AN ATHLETIC TRAINER'S GUIDE TO

SPORTS NUTRITION

Damon Amato, MS, LAT, CSCS
Head Athletic Trainer
Lowell High School
Lowell, Massachusetts

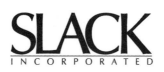

SLACK
INCORPORATED

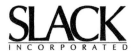

SLACK Incorporated
6900 Grove Road
Thorofare, NJ 08086 USA
856-848-1000   Fax: 856-848-6091
www.Healio.com/books
© 2019 by SLACK Incorporated

Senior Vice President: Stephanie Arasim Portnoy
Vice President, Editorial: Jennifer Kilpatrick
Vice President, Marketing: Michelle Gatt
Acquisitions Editor: Brien Cummings
Managing Editor: Allegra Tiver
Creative Director: Thomas Cavallaro
Cover Artist: Christine Seabo
Project Editor: Dani Malady

The procedures and practices described in this publication should be implemented in a manner consistent with the professional standards set for the circumstances that apply in each specific situation. Every effort has been made to confirm the accuracy of the information presented and to correctly relate generally accepted practices. The authors, editors, and publisher cannot accept responsibility for errors or exclusions or for the outcome of the material presented herein. There is no expressed or implied warranty of this book or information imparted by it. Care has been taken to ensure that drug selection and dosages are in accordance with currently accepted/recommended practice. Off-label uses of drugs may be discussed. Due to continuing research, changes in government policy and regulations, and various effects of drug reactions and interactions, it is recommended that the reader carefully review all materials and literature provided for each drug, especially those that are new or not frequently used. Some drugs or devices in this publication have clearance for use in a restricted research setting by the Food and Drug and Administration or FDA. Each professional should determine the FDA status of any drug or device prior to use in their practice.

Any review or mention of specific companies or products is not intended as an endorsement by the author or publisher.

SLACK Incorporated uses a review process to evaluate submitted material. Prior to publication, educators or clinicians provide important feedback on the content that we publish. We welcome feedback on this work.

Library of Congress Cataloging-in-Publication Data

Names: Amato, Damon, author.
Title: An athletic trainer's guide to sports nutrition / Damon Amato.
Description: Thorofare, [N.J.] : SLACK Incorporated, 2018. | Includes
   bibliographical references and index.
Identifiers: LCCN 2018026471 (print) | LCCN 2018027760 (ebook) | ISBN
   9781630914257 (epub) | ISBN 9781630914264 (web) | ISBN 9781630914240 (pbk.
   : alk. paper)
Subjects: | MESH: Sports Nutritional Physiological Phenomena
Classification: LCC RA784 (ebook) | LCC RA784 (print) | NLM QT 263 | DDC
   613.202/4796--dc23
LC record available at https://lccn.loc.gov/2018026471

Printed in the United States of America.

Last digit is print number: 10   9   8   7   6   5   4   3   2   1

AN ATHLETIC TRAINER'S GUIDE TO

SPORTS
NUTRITION

DEDICATION

This text is dedicated to my mom, who sacrificed and worked tirelessly her entire life in constant care of her family. I miss her every day.

CONTENTS

ACKNOWLEDGMENTS

This text would not have been possible without the love and support of my wife, Larissa. She was incredibly patient and caring during this process. It was her suggestion, in fact, that I take this text on to get me to stop complaining about the poor quality of other texts that I was using to teach in order to provide medical professionals with a more readable script that is applicable in the field. I would also like to thank all the expert contributors who graciously devoted their own time to write a section or full chapter in this text. Their dedication to their respective fields truly elevates the quality of this text.

ABOUT THE AUTHOR

Damon Amato, MS, LAT, CSCS is an Athletic Trainer, Strength Coach, and Nutritionist with 13 years' experience in the field. With a broad knowledge base in the athletic domain, Damon has trained individuals from stay-at-home moms to mixed martial artists to college team sport athletes. His passion for helping athletes and practitioners alike flows through multiple disciplines, gathering expert resources in all facets of athleticism. With a master's degree in applied nutrition and a certification through the National Strength and Conditioning Association, Damon spends most of his time helping high school athletes as the Head Athletic Trainer at the largest public high school in Massachusetts and also teaching performance nutrition courses at the college level.

Contributing Authors

Jennifer L. Gaudiani, MD, CEDS, FAED (Chapter 4)
Founder and Medical Director
Gaudiani Clinic
Denver, Colorado

John Kiefer, MS (Chapter 6, Creatine)
Oakland, California

Karl Nadolsky, DO (Chapter 9, Diabetes)
Board Certified, Endocrinology, Diabetes & Metabolism
Diplomate, American Board of Obesity Medicine
Assistant Clinical Professor of Medicine
Michigan State University College of Human Medicine
Grand Rapids, Michigan

Stacy Sims, BSc, MSc, PhD (Chapter 5)
Te Huataki Waiora Faculty
Health, Sport and Human Performance
Adams Centre for High Performance
University of Waikato
Hamilton, New Zealand

PREFACE

I see this textbook being a valuable resource for athletic trainers. The current athletic trainer curriculum does not devote nearly enough time to the importance of nutrition, especially since athletes ask athletic trainers about it all the time. It is a subject that I feel is much underappreciated but is of paramount importance. It was written in a tone that can be easily read and understood by medical professionals, yet in-depth enough to create a solid understanding of how the body really works, and easy enough to then pass on the information to athletes in order to help them eat optimally based on their specific sport, goal, and situation.

Giving a physiology background is necessary to lay the foundation for understanding why certain recommendations in the book are given; however, I only present what is necessary to understand concepts of performance nutrition and do not go into more details about human physiology that are not pertinent for athletic trainers to understand while advising athletes.

I have included in the table of contents what I think are the most important subjects for an athletic trainer to be educated in, and how I teach my students. Most athletes just want to know basics of how to eat, when to eat, and what to eat. For the vast majority of them, that information is sufficient. The nuances of nutrient timing and energy balance are the subjects that require the most attention, and athletic trainers will need the most education on those subjects specifically because that is where most of the bad information is sourced from in the current research.

Introduction

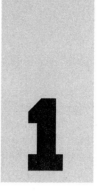

WHO IS THIS BOOK FOR?

This book should be used for athletic trainers in courses that are evidence based, are scientific, and concern clinical application of nutrition in order to improve health or performance. Physical therapists, physicians, strength and conditioning coaches, and personal trainers will also find this text useful.

In today's climate of health care practitioners, we are all expected to be experts in all aspects of our respective fields by the general population. Over the past decade, physical therapists have evolved to higher degrees, dry needling, and spine manipulation. Athletic trainers now have employment opportunities in the military, with law enforcement, at the corporate level, and as physician extenders. With all of these new certifications and responsibility comes a need for further education in order to provide proper care not only to athletes or injured individuals, but also to those seeking to just look and feel better. Nutrition education is paramount for reaching those goals.

Athletic training is widely regarded as a clinical health care profession, and the education of athletic trainers should be treated as such. In the various settings that athletic trainers may be employed in, it is extremely likely that at some point, an athlete, client, customer, soldier, or officer wants to know what to eat, when to eat, how much to eat, and other more complicated questions. Athletic trainers should be held accountable for knowing the answer to these questions to a certain degree, and they will have a greater knowledge base after reading this text. We are all athletes in some aspect, so for the purposes of simplicity, we will use only the terms *practitioner* and *athlete* when discussing individuals.

Amato D. *An Athletic Trainer's Guide to Sports Nutrition* (pp 1-2).
© 2019 SLACK Incorporated.

Health care professionals should use this textbook as a guide for laying the foundation for their own education and as a way to extrapolate information necessary to help the athletes under their care. There is no one perfect diet, and practitioners will learn from this text how to treat each athlete as an individual with individual needs that may vary from person to person.

Diet Influences

Food preferences reveal a lot about who we are as a person. It can change based on interactions with family, friends, or teammates, and really shapes habits later in life. Convenience and cost also play a large role in the food choices that we make, so it is easy to see that there are a variety of factors that can influence the current eating habits of an athlete. In many cases, learning to adopt new and healthier habits can be the most difficult task a practitioner can have when treating an athlete.

Businesses spend about $9.7 billion annually to market and advertise food products, oftentimes aggressively and dishonestly. As you will see in a later chapter, cereal was only adopted as a breakfast food because of the marketing and political sway of the company that created corn flakes, not because of any scientific research to show that eating cereal in the morning is of any nutritional benefit.

Social factors have become increasingly important to the younger generation as well. Posting meals on social media as well as pressure to join in at family events, office parties, or team dinners can put a lot of peer pressure on someone, even with a lot of willpower. It is these influences that, for better or worse, can mold a person's eating habits whether they consciously choose to or not. With so much knowledge and contrasting opinions at everyone's fingertips, it becomes increasing difficult to have your own plan that you want to stick to without having someone quickly look up your food choices on the internet and come up with multiple reasons why you should not make the choices that you have. Thankfully, this text will provide the tools and knowledge base to make informed decisions about everyday food choices. Learning about nutrition makes us all more informed and leads to more educated discussions on varying or subjective opinions.

It is essential to have at least a basic understanding of biology, anatomy, physiology, and chemistry in order to understand nutrition adequately. This chapter will introduce fundamental yet important anatomy, processes, concepts, and terms related to human nutrition that will provide a basis to understand more difficult concepts explained later in this text. Certain cell structures such as mitochondria and muscle cells are as important as the different classifications of nutrients (protein, fat, carbohydrate, vitamins, minerals, water), and processes like the Krebs cycle, electron transport chain, and glucose fatty acid cycle are crucial in understanding how to train athletes to better utilize different energy systems.

In addition to understanding the composition of nutrients and the processes they govern, it will be important to understand how certain processes correlate with each other. Certain hormones like ghrelin and cortisol have diurnal rhythms that present an environment that make the composition of meals more important, while eating meals with specific macronutrient compositions can create an internal milieu that could be very beneficial or very negative, depending on its context. These concepts will provide the practitioner with the tools necessary to advise athletes.

Basics of
Human Nutrition

2

Key Takeaways

* Structure and function of mitochondria in relation to muscle and liver cells will elucidate how glucose metabolism works.
* The glucose fatty acid cycle is a process that describes the competition between carbohydrate and fatty acids to be used as energy substrates.
* Specific hunger hormones can regulate how nutrients are converted.
* Glucose is absolutely necessary for only 2 tasks: excessive glycogen storage and excessive fat storage.

Cell Structure

This is a cell (Figure 2-1), and for our purposes, it can be either a liver cell or a muscle cell because those cells are where we store glycogen, the storage form of glucose. Within this cell are several cell structures called *organelles*. The cell contains a plasma membrane, cytoplasm, mitochondria, ribosomes, lysosomes, endoplasmic reticulum, Golgi apparatus, and the nuclear envelope. The cell can be divided into the nucleus and the cytoplasm. The plasma membrane is composed of proteins, phospholipids, cholesterol, other lipids, and carbs.

More detail of the entire cell structure is beyond the scope of this text, and we are mostly interested in the interplay of the mitochondria as it relates to metabolic pathways for energy.

Amato D. *An Athletic Trainer's Guide to Sports Nutrition (pp 5-28).*
© 2019 SLACK Incorporated.

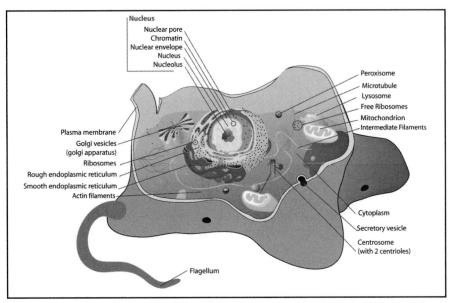

Figure 2-1. Cell structure. (Reprinted from https://commons.wikimedia.org/wiki/File%3AAnimal_cell_structure_en.svg. By LadyofHats (Mariana Ruiz) [Public domain], via Wikimedia Commons from Wikimedia Commons.)

Mitochondria

The mitochondria are the "power house" of the cell membrane and are found in almost every cell in the human body. Mitochondria vary in size, shape, and density depending on where they are in the body, and they generate adenosine triphosphate (ATP), the energy currency in the body. They are mostly found in areas of organelles with high-energy demands such as the nucleus or near contractile myofibril in muscle cells. Mitochondria contain 2 lipid/protein bilayers called the *outer membrane* and *inner membrane*, as seen in Figure 2-2.

It also provides a barrier for the mitochondrial matrix, which is concentrated with enzymes involved in energy nutrient oxidation and DNA.

METABOLIC PROCESSES

Krebs Cycle

The Krebs cycle (also called *TCA cycle* or *citric acid cycle*, depending on the textbook) is a series of 7 chemical reactions where **oxaloacetate** is regenerated. The results of these reactions are the reduced cofactors that will then transfer to the electron transport chain. These include nicotinamide adenine dinucleotide (NADH) and flavin adenine dinucleotide (FADH2), which are the reduced forms of NAD+ and

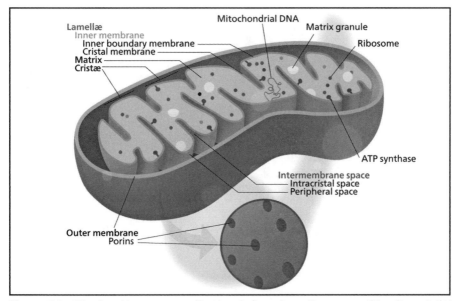

Figure 2-2. Mitochondria structure. (Reprinted from https://commons.wikimedia.org/wiki/File%3AMitochondrion_structure.svg. By Kelvinsong; modified by Sowlos (Own work based on: Mitochondrion mini.svg) [CC BY-SA 3.0 (https://creativecommons.org/licenses/by-sa/3.0)], via Wikimedia Commons from Wikimedia Commons.)

FAD, among other reactions. One important point to note is that ATP is generated anaerobically in one reaction of glycolysis; this is the sole source of ATP for erythrocytes or red blood cells, which do not have mitochondria. This is not the case for most cells as their ATP is generated through **oxidative phosphorylation** by the electron transport chain (Figure 2-3).

Electron Transport Chain

The electron transport chain occurs in the mitochondrial inner membrane. Oxygen is needed for the electron transport chain. NADH and FADH2 transfer electrons to the electron transport chain. NADH is free-floating throughout the mitochondrial matrix and cytosol and may need to diffuse to the electron transport chain depending on its location. FADH2 is bound to enzymes in the inner membrane, which is thought to be immediately available to the electron transport chain. With the electron transport chain, 3 ATP molecules for each NADH and 2 ATP molecules for each FADH2 are created (Figure 2-4).

Glucose Fatty Acid Cycle

The glucose fatty acid cycle (or *Randle cycle*) is a process that describes the competition between carbs and fatty acids to be used as energy substrates.[1] Randle and Morgan[2] conducted research in the 1960s investigating the inhibitory effect of fat

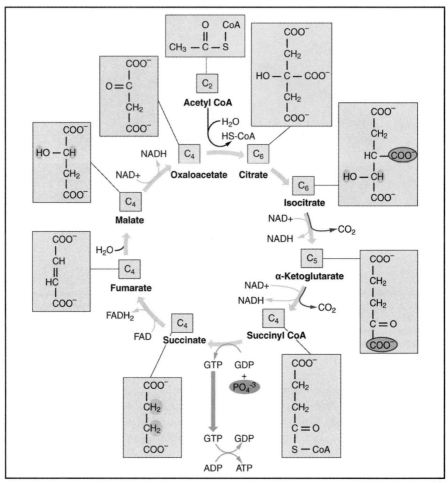

Figure 2-3. Simplified Krebs cycle. (Reprinted from https://commons.wikimedia.org/wiki/File%3A2507_The_Krebs_Cycle.jpg. By OpenStax College [CC BY 3.0 (http://creativecommons.org/licenses/by/3.0)], via Wikimedia Commons from Wikimedia Commons.)

metabolism on carb metabolism. They used heart and diaphragm muscle from rats in test tubes, where they took live samples of tissue, snap froze them, and then added fat to it to see what would happen. The tissue incubated did not burn carbs. They postulated that fat inhibits it because of pathways identified for carb metabolism. This theory stood without being challenged for 30 years as a switch for carb/fat metabolism that happens in all tissues in the human body. However, that is not correct. Rat tissue is certainly a confounding factor when extrapolating this information for humans, but that is not the problem with the methodology. The larger problem is that the tissue being tested was heart and diaphragm muscle, not skeletal muscle. Heart and diaphragm muscle do not have glycogen, the storage form of glucose and essentially the most important aspect of the research. Muscle glycogen plays a major role in what gets burned as energy.

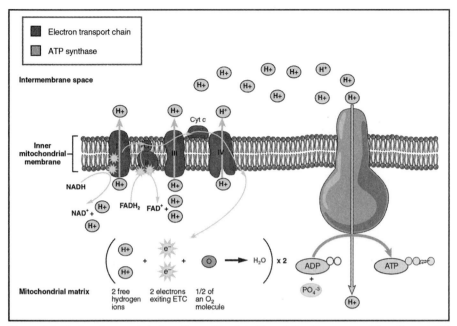

Figure 2-4. Electron transport chain pathway. (Reprinted from https://commons.wikimedia.org/wiki/ File%3A2508_The_Electron_Transport_Chain.jpg. By OpenStax College [CC BY 3.0 (http://creative-commons.org/licenses/by/3.0)], via Wikimedia Commons from Wikimedia Commons.)

The 1990s research was in Scandinavia, where the investigators took grad students, cannulated their femoral arteries, infused emulsified lipid solutions, got them to exercise, and, during exercise, took skeletal muscle biopsies.[3] Not only is this interesting as it was a more "real world" strategy, but clearly it would be difficult to find volunteers for such a study. From this research, they could conclude through plasma glucose uptake and fatty acid oxidation, "we discovered that a large proportion of the fatty acids are synthesized from other sources."[4]

Another study from Odland et al[1] said it is the entry of fat into the mitochondria, not so much glycolysis, that is important because that produces large amounts of malonyl-CoA, which is formed from acetyl-CoA during fatty acid synthesis.[5] In rats, there was great evidence in the Randle study. In humans, it does not hold true. Rats produce thousands of times as much malonyl-CoA than humans do. The metabolism of fatty acids and carbs results in products that can specifically inhibit the catabolism of the other.

Glucose Transporters

Insulin is thought of as the key that opens the lock to get sugar and fat cells into muscle, but it does not do the actual work. That is performed by glucose transporters (GLUTs). We currently know of 14 of these: GLUT1 through GLUT14. GLUT5 actually transports fructose into the liver, while others hamper the transport

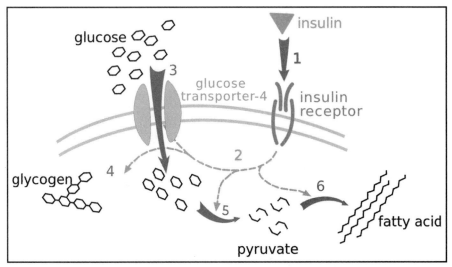

Figure 2-5. GLUT pathway. (Reprinted from https://commons.wikimedia.org/wiki/File%3AInsulin_glucose_metabolism_ZP.svg. By XcepticZP at en.wikipedia [Public domain], via Wikimedia Commons from Wikimedia Commons.)

of glucose. GLUTs 1 through 4 actually do transport glucose to muscle cells and, of these, GLUT4 and GLUT12 are perhaps the most important.

When not active, GLUT4 proteins sit within the inner membrane of the cell, doing nothing. Once insulin comes in contact with a cell containing them, the GLUTs translocate to the surface of the cell where they adhere to glucose molecules and move them into the interior of the cell.[6] The cell then uses the glucose as energy or stores it within the cell (Figure 2-5).

Insulin sensitivity is heavily referenced when describing whether someone is prediabetic. It relates how reactive a cell is to the insulin-triggered translocation of GLUT4 and GLUT12 proteins from the interior of the cell to the exterior. If cells do not react to insulin or more than normal insulin is secreted for GLUTs to move to the cell surface, the person is deemed "insulin insensitive." This excess secretion of insulin takes a toll on the pancreas where it comes from, and that can eventually cause type II diabetes. Insulin resistance happens when they do not move at all.

Two tissues contain high amounts of GLUT4: striated muscle cells and fat cells. When someone has high insulin sensitivity, both fat and muscle cells are able to store as glucose or triaglycerol, the storage form of fat. When you become insulin-resistant, neither cell is able to do that. It is your body's last-ditch effort to keep itself robust before becoming unhealthy. It is these facts that beg the question, is obesity the cause of disease or a symptom of it?

NUTRIENT CONVERSION

Proteins, fats, and carbs may all go to the same place, but they do not end up performing the same actions on the body. In fact, each one has the potential to be converted into something else that the human body can utilize for a different function.

Liver and fat cells will turn glucose directly into fatty acids through a process called **de novo lipogenesis**.[7-18] That process becomes very energy expensive, so the actual amount of glucose that gets converted into fatty acids is only about 5%.[14,19,20]

In contrast, fructose, another monosaccharide, can contribute significantly to de novo lipogenesis when ingested in large amounts. The body regulates massive feedings with glucose through a rate-limited step that prevents pure glucose from sparking lipogenesis.,[21] but fructose can create unlimited byproducts that lead to the accumulation of fat.[4,12,22]

Where carbs contribute most significantly and efficiently to fat storage is through conversion into glycerol complexes.[14,23-25] A triaglycerol molecule, the body's most abundant form of stored fat, has a glycerol backbone connected to 3 fatty acids. That is why glucose and fructose can easily be converted into glycerol for the storage of more fat.

Recent research has shown that the chemical **myostatin** also plays a large role in whether humans tend to store or burn body fat. Myostatin is a growth factor that regulates the size of muscles beginning in early embryonic development and continues throughout life. Myostatin acts by inhibiting the growth of muscles; it prevents them from growing too large. When myostatin is found in higher than normal concentrations, muscle mass is decreased.[26-34] There is also evidence that it has been associated with sarcopenia.[35]

The muscle-building and fat-burning effects of **human growth hormone** (GH) are thought to be caused by GH's interference with myostatin function,[36] and **cortisol** levels may be associated with higher concentrations of myostatin, which could be destructive to muscle.[37] Elevated myostatin levels have also been found in astronauts who suffer from muscle disuse atrophy.[31,38] The most compelling subject regarding myostatin is the difference in fat and muscle tissue mass between males and females.[39]

When athletes eat a diet regimen that is in a caloric deficit, increases in concentration of myostatin in muscles are seen and can lead to muscle wasting.[40] It is for this reason that the most common response from practitioners would be to eat more protein to spare muscle wasting; however, this is only one mechanism of correction that does not fully address the problem. What is more important is identifying the proper hormonal milieu that would be most likely to spare muscle tissue during a caloric deficit. This means knowing the athlete's medical history (type I diabetes, gluten allergy, etc) and tailoring a regiment based on what fits his or her lifestyle.

Hormone Connection

There are 2 important hormones that regulate insulin: **hormone-sensitive lipase** (HSL) and **lipoprotein lipase** (LPL). Insulin itself is a very important hormone that is not well understood with regard to energy utilization and blood sugar regulation, but that is not all insulin does.

Insulin stimulates muscle to build new protein[41] and it inhibits lipolysis, the breakdown of fat.[42] This is very important in relation to the interaction of HSL and LPL. HSL is responsible for breaking triglycerides down into free fatty acids that can mobilize out of fat cells and get used for energy, but insulin downregulates HSL in fat cells at the same time it downregulates LPL in muscle cells. This means that large releases on insulin inhibit utilization of free fatty acids as energy, and the body must rely on glucose in the blood for the most part.

LPL does the opposite of HSL by pulling fatty acids into fat cells to increase their size, as well as assisting to increase intramuscular triaglycerol levels, though the specific mechanism is still up for debate.[43]

We can also use stores of muscle and liver glycogen as energy as well, but insulin also inhibits access to muscle glycogen stores. That is why you sometimes see marathon runners "hit the wall" during a race. *Hitting the wall* is a term used when a runner completely runs out of energy and must stop activity because he or she simply cannot continue. The theory used to be that this happens because the runner's muscle and liver glycogen stores are empty and they lack any energy stores; however, this has been proven to be false.[44] Runners still have plenty of muscle glycogen left, but they are still unable to continue.

The reason is not due to lack of muscle glycogen, it is due to the lack of access to muscle glycogen. This happens because every one-half mile or so, the runners continue to ingest fast-acting carbs such as gels or sports drinks, which trigger a high release of insulin. Insulin inhibits lipolysis and glycogen utilization at the same time, preventing the runner from being able to effectively use much of anything for energy at such an intense rate. While these molecules ingested from exogenous sources enter the blood stream relatively quickly, they can only provide a minute amount of energy compared to the amount being expended during a race, and eventually the stomach will require more time than is needed to process enough carbs into the blood stream in order to be expended. Large influxes of amino acids from protein can also cause insulin release. Leucine, an important amino acid, can cause a large insulin release independent of other sources as well.[45]

With HSL being downregulated via lower-scale insulin release, it becomes difficult to get fat out of fat cells. That is why when cells are covered in insulin, both LPL (which pulls fatty acids into cells) and insulin—released in heavy doses when you eat most carbs—partitions more fat into storage than when you eat pure fat. Glucose is absolutely necessary for only 2 tasks: excessive glycogen storage and excessive fat storage.

Hunger Hormones

Ghrelin

Hunger and appetite are regulated by the endocrine system. Exactly how that works has not been completely elucidated yet, however. We originally thought that a rapid rise in insulin, followed by an associated fall in blood sugar, stimulated appetite, which would in turn stimulate overeating. This theory is well explained by the South Beach Diet, however incorrect it may be.[46]

This mechanism for overeating was studied multiple times and has since not panned out as scientific fact.[47,48] Unfortunately, for a long time, there was no alternative explanation. This changed in 1999 with the discovery of the hormone ghrelin.[49,50]

Ghrelin was the first hormone discovered to directly stimulate hunger in humans.[51] It is produced in the gut, making it difficult to associate originally because there are so many different pathways and organisms moving around at all times.[52-63] Since its discovery, we now know several properties about ghrelin, including its potential ability to regulate body weight. Since 1999, many studies have been done to elucidate all of the properties of ghrelin. Recently, a review of some of these studies was put together by one of this text's contributors, John Kiefer, as well as similar properties of leptin in the next section. These are summarized as follows:

* It stimulates GH release in humans[49,56,64-73] and is possibly the most potent stimulator of GH release in the body.[74] A few conflicting results exist.[74,75]
* Higher concentrations directly increase hunger.[50,51,76-82]
* Levels fall after meal ingestion.[50,77,78,81,83-89]
* Directly related to body mass[65,90-104]; the more fat mass, the lower the levels of ghrelin.
* Higher levels are found in women.[83,92,105]
* It has a possible role in male sex hormone production.[106-108]

These properties of ghrelin position it high on the list of body weight regulators,[51,109-111] especially since it signals overall fat stores and nutritional status of the body (i.e., the more fat you possess and the more you eat, the lower your levels of ghrelin).[82,91,112-115]

Ghrelin appears as a direct link between the gut and the brain,[116-119] and there is even evidence that it causes a timing effect for meal ingestion during the day.[120] It may also trigger a deeper state of sleep in humans.[120] Even the success of gastric bypass surgery to reduce weight seems to be related to ghrelin secretion—or a lack thereof.[94,121,122]

This is a hormone requiring particular consideration in any type of diet, whether you are a serious athlete or not,[122] and it is definitely a hormone we are going to target for manipulation.

Leptin

Leptin is a critical hormone in terms of the complications of obesity and weight loss. In 1994, a mutation in a specific mouse gene led to massive obesity and type II diabetes.[122] This mutated gene was appropriately called the *Ob gene.*

Normal mice without the defective gene produce a hormone that, when administered to mice with the mutation, causes them to lose weight, decrease body fat, and suppresses appetite. The administration of this hormone even reverses the symptoms of type II diabetes.[123-125] It was called *leptin* after the Greek *leptós*, which, quite appropriately in this case, means "thin."

More importantly, humans also produce leptin,[122] and those with the defective Ob gene are massively obese.[126,127] This mutation is extremely rare in humans. In fact, it is nearly nonexistent,[128] but leptin is still an important weight-control hormone for "normal" people.

Leptin is produced mainly in the white fat cells of the body. The more fat cells you have and the larger they get, the more leptin is produced.[129-145] As a result, leptin levels correlate with the amount of fat stored, although some researchers differ on this.[146,147] Even in extremely skinny people, leptin levels are associated with the amount of body fat present.[142]

There's also evidence of subcutaneous fat as the major leptin producer.[134,137-139,143,148-151] A higher-than-normal amount of fat gives you an incredible advantage when you start your weight loss program because of the high levels of leptin produced. A summary of the properties of leptin are as follows:

* Increases metabolism[123-125,152-155]
* Specifically increases fat burning[156-165]
* Prevents the formation and storage of fat[156,161,164-169]
* Women possess higher levels[133,134,144,170-174] although there is some discrepancy[175]
* Regulates several hormones in the brain to decrease appetite and food intake[155,176-199] and may independently cause decreased food intake[182,200-203]
* Reproductive effects: improves fertility,[204-211] causes puberty to occur at a younger age in females with elevated levels,[210,212-226] and low levels inhibit the onset of puberty[216,219,223,227]
* Appears to decrease desire for sweets[228-231]
* Increases the activity and production of immune system cells[232,233]
* Production decreases with age regardless of changes in fat mass[145,223,227]

When leptin levels get low, you get hungry and your body stops mobilizing fat from fat stores to burn. When you are dieting, the situation gets even worse because most diets decrease levels of leptin,[141,234] making it difficult to maintain weight loss. The low leptin levels caused by dieting also make it very easy to regain the weight.[234-236] To neglect all consideration of leptin's action when designing a diet is absurd since nearly all researchers seem to agree that leptin is essential for weight maintenance.[203,211,224,237]

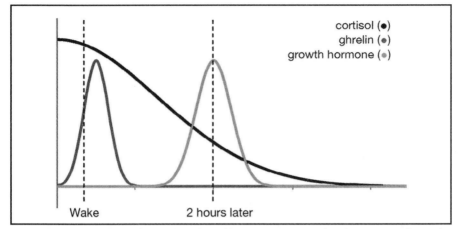

Figure 2-6. Morning chart of diurnal rhythm of hormones. (Reprinted with permission from John Kiefer, http://athlete.io/.)

Cortisol

Cortisol is a hormone released by the adrenal glands during times of stress. It can be tested via blood, saliva, or urine, which is important as humans can develop a condition called Cushing's syndrome, which involves having too much of the hormone, or Addison's disease, which is caused by having too little.

For the average individual, upon waking or thereabouts, levels of the cortisol reach a high point for the day. Cortisol elevates naturally through the night[225,226] and peaks upon waking.[225,238] Cortisol is catabolic, meaning it breaks down a more complex material in the body for a different use. In this context, cortisol is important because it is a normal process associated with resistance training. Releasing glucose from glycogen stores is also catabolic, as is releasing fat from fat cells.

A graph of the important diurnal rhythms of certain hormones is shown here. Based on these, we can see how the timing of certain macronutrients could affect these patterns (Figure 2-6).

CONCLUSION

An entire text could be filled with important hormones that regulate weight, weight loss, weight gain, mood, and other interesting developments in the human body; however, this chapter's intent was to bring to light the most important of those hormones and processes so that practitioners may better understand what is necessary and leave the more complicated issues to biochemists. Understanding how basic hormones interact on bodily functions—especially hunger—will allow practitioners to better convey recommendations to athletes.

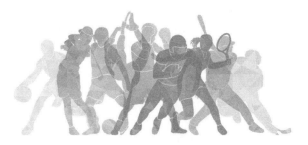

DEFINITIONS

Oxaloacetate: An intermediate of the Krebs cycle and the stage immediately prior to the formation of pyruvate

Oxidative phosphorylation: The process in cell metabolism by which respiratory enzymes in the mitochondria synthesize ATP from andinorganic phosphate (ADP) during the oxidation of NADH by molecular oxygen

De novo lipogenesis: The biochemical process of synthesizing fatty acids from acetyl-CoA subunits that are produced from a number of different pathways within the cell, most commonly carbohydrate catabolism

Myostatin: A protein produced and released by muscle cells that acts on their autocrine function to inhibit muscle cell growth and differentiation

Human growth hormone: A peptide hormone that stimulates growth, cell reproduction, and cell regeneration in humans

Cortisol: A steroid-based hormone synthesized by cholesterol involved in the regulation of metabolism in the cells that helps us regulate stress within the body

Hormone-sensitive lipase: An enzyme that catalyzes the release of fatty acids from adipose tissues

Lipoprotein lipase: An enzyme that plays a key role in breaking down triglycerides present in chylomicrons and very low-density lipoprotein particles, releasing their fatty acids for entry into tissue cells

REFERENCES

1. Odland LM, Heigenhauser GJ, Lopaschuk GD, Spriet LL. Human skeletal muscle malonyl-CoA at rest and during prolonged submaximal exercise. *Am J Physiol.* 1996:270;E541-E544.
2. Randle PJ, Morgan HE. Regulation of glucose uptake by muscle. *Biochem J.* 1964:93;652-665.
3. Hargreaves M, Kiens B, Richter EA. Effect of increased plasma free fatty acid concentrations on muscle metabolism in exercising men. *J Appl Physiol.* 1991:70;194-201.
4. Collins JM, Neville MJ, Pinnick KE, et al. De novo lipogenesis in the differentiating human adipocyte can provide all fatty acids necessary for maturation. *J Lipid Res.* 2011;52(9):1683-1692.

5. Collins JM, Neville MJ, Hoppa MB, Frayn KN. De novo lipogenesis and stearoyl-CoA desaturase are coordinately regulated in the human adipocyte and protect against palmitate-induced cell injury. *J Biol Chem*. 2010;285(9):6044-6052.

6. Yang J, Yujing C, Burkhardt B, et al. Leucine metabolism in regulation of insulin secretion from pancreatic beta cells. *Nutr Rev*. 2010;68(5):270-279.

7. Wilke MS, French MA, Goh YK, Ryan EA, Jones PJ, Clandinin MT. Synthesis of specific fatty acids contributes to VLDL-triacylglycerol composition in humans with and without type 2 diabetes. *Diabetologia*. 2009;52(8):1628-1637.

8. Roberts R, Hodson L, Dennis AL, et al. Markers of de novo lipogenesis in adipose tissue: associations with small adipocytes and insulin sensitivity in humans. *Diabetologia*. 2009;52(5):882-890.

9. Chong MF, Hodson L, Bickerton AS, et al. Parallel activation of de novo lipogenesis and stearoyl-CoA desaturase activity after 3 d of high-carbohydrate feeding. *Am J Clin Nutr*. 2008;87(4):817-823.

10. Strawford A, Antelo F, Christiansen M, Hellerstein MK. Adipose tissue triglyceride turnover, de novo lipogenesis, and cell proliferation in humans measured with 2H2O. *Am J Physiol Endocrinol Metab*. 2004;286(4):E577-E588.

11. Minehira K, Bettschart V, Vidal H, et al. Effect of carbohydrate overfeeding on whole body and adipose tissue metabolism in humans. *Obes Res*. 2003;11(9):1096-1103.

12. Guo ZK, Cella LK, Baum C, Ravussin E, Schoeller DA. De novo lipogenesis in adipose tissue of lean and obese women: application of deuterated water and isotope ratio mass spectrometry. *Int J Obes Relat Metab Disord*. 2000;24(7):932-937.

13. Hellerstein MK, Neese RA, Schwarz JM. Model for measuring absolute rates of hepatic de novo lipogenesis and reesterification of free fatty acids. *Am J Physiol*. 1993;265(5 Pt 1):E814-E820.

14. Shrago E, Spennetta T. The carbon pathway for lipogenesis in isolated adipocytes from rat, guinea pig, and human adipose tissue. *Am J Clin Nutr*. 1976;29(5):540-545.

15. Bray GA. Lipogenesis in human adipose tissue: some effects of nibbling and gorging. *J Clin Invest*. 1972;51(3):537-548.

16. Mellati AM, Beck JC, Dupre J, Rubinstein D. Conversion of glucose to lipid by human adipose tissue in vitro. *Metabolism*. 1970;19(11):988-994.

17. Hellerstein MK, Schwarz JM, Neese RA. Regulation of hepatic de novo lipogenesis in humans. *Annu Rev Nutr*. 1996;16:523-557.

18. Mayes PA. Intermediary metabolism of fructose. *Am J Clin Nutr*. 1993;58(5 Suppl):754S-765S.

19. Goldrick RB, McLoughlin GM. Lipolysis and lipogenesis from glucose in human fat cells of different sizes. Effects of insulin, epinephrine, and theophylline. *J Clin Invest*. 1970;49(6):1213-1223.

20. Maruhama Y. Conversion of ingested carbohydrate-14C into glycerol and fatty acids of serum triglyceride in patients with myocardial infarction. *Metabolism*. 1970;19(12):1085-1093.

21. Schwarz JM, Neese RA, Schakleton C, Hellerstein MK. De novo lipogenesis during fasting and oral fructose ingestion in lean and obese hyperinsulinemic subjects. *Diabetes*. 1993;42(suppl):A39.

22. Schwarz J-M, Neese RA, Turner SM, Nguyen C, Hellerstein MK. Effect of fructose ingestion on glucose production (GP) and de novo lipogenesis (DNL) in normal and hyperinsulinemic obese humans. *Diabetes*. 1994;43(suppl):52A.

23. Barter PJ, Nestel PJ, Carroll KF. Precursors of plasma triglyceride fatty acid in humans. Effects of glucose consumption, clofibrate administration, and alcoholic fatty liver. *Metabolism*. 1972;21(2):117-124.

24. Timmerman KL, Lee JL, Dreyer HC, et al. Insulin stimulates human skeletal muscle protein synthesis via an indirect mechanism involving endothelial-dependent vasodilation and mammalian target of rapamycin complex 1 signaling. *J Clin Endocrinol Metab.* 2010;95(8):3848-3857.

25. Kersten S. Mechanisms of nutritional and hormonal regulation of lipogenesis. *EMBO Rep.* 2001;2(4):282-286.

26. Joulia D, Bernardi H, Garandel V, Rabenoelina F, Vernus B, Cabello G. Mechanisms involved in the inhibition of myoblast proliferation and differentiation by myostatin. *Exp Cell Res.* 2003;286(2):263-275.

27. Zimmers TA, Davies MV, Koniaris LG, et al. Induction of cachexia in mice by systemically administered myostatin. *Science.* 2002;296(5572):1486-1488.

28. Rios R, Carneiro I, Arce VM, Devesa J. Myostatin is an inhibitor of myogenic differentiation. *Am J Physiol Cell Physiol.* 2002;282(5):C993-C999.

29. Reardon KA, Davis J, Kapsa RM, Choong P, Byrne E. Myostatin, insulin-like growth factor-1, and leukemia inhibitory factor mRNAs are upregulated in chronic human disuse muscle atrophy. *Muscle Nerve.* 2001;24(7):893-899.

30. Taylor WE, Bhasin S, Artaza J, et al. Myostatin inhibits cell proliferation and protein synthesis in C2C12 muscle cells. *Am J Physiol Endocrinol Metab.* 2001;280(2):E221-E228.

31. Thomas M, Langley B, Berry C, et al. Myostatin, a negative regulator of muscle growth, functions by inhibiting myoblast proliferation. *J Biol Chem.* 2000;275(51):40235-40243.

32. Kirk S, Oldham J, Kambadur R, Sharma M, Dobbie P, Bass J. Myostatin regulation during skeletal muscle regeneration. *J Cell Physiol.* 2000;184(3):356-363.

33. Yarasheski KE, Bhasin S, Sinha-Hikim I, Pak-Loduca J, Gonzalez-Cadavid NF. Serum myostatin-immunoreactive protein is increased in 60-92 year old women and men with muscle wasting. *J Nutr Health Aging.* 2002;6(5):343-348.

34. Liu W, Thomas SG, Asa SL, Gonzalez-Cadavid N, Bhasin S, Ezzat S. Myostatin is a skeletal muscle target of growth hormone anabolic action. *J Clin Endocrinol Metab.* 2003;88(11):5490-5496.

35. Ma K, Mallidis C, Bhasin S, et al. Glucocorticoid-induced skeletal muscle atrophy is associated with upregulation of myostatin gene expression. *Am J Physiol Endocrinol Metab.* 2003;285(2):E363-E371.

36. Zachwieja JJ, Smith SR, Sinha-Hikim I, Gonzalez-Cadavid N, Bhasin S. Plasma myostatin-immunoreactive protein is increased after prolonged bed rest with low-dose T3 administration. *J Gravit Physiol.* 1999;6(2):11-15.

37. McMahon CD, Popovic L, Jeanplong F, et al. Sexual dimorphism is associated with decreased expression of processed myostatin in males. *Am J Physiol Endocrinol Metab.* 2003;284(2):E377-E381.

38. Jeanplong F, Bass JJ, Smith HK, et al. Prolonged underfeeding of sheep increases myostatin and myogenic regulatory factor Myf-5 in skeletal muscle while IGF-I and myogenin are repressed. *J Endocrinol.* 2003;176(3):425-437.

39. Agatston A. *The South Beach Diet.* New York, NY: Random House; 2003.

40. Geiselman PJ. Sugar-induced hyperphagia: is hyperinsulinemia, hypoglycemia, or any other factor a "necessary" condition? *Appetite.* 1988;11(Suppl 1):26-34.

41. Madsen K, Pedersen PK, Rose P. Carbohydrate supercompensation and muscle glycogen utilization during exhaustive running in highly trained athletes. *Eur J Appl Physiol Occup Physiol.* 1990;61(5-6):467-472.

42. Barnard RJ, Youngren JF. Regulation of glucose transport in skeletal muscle. *FASEB J.* 1992;6(14):3238-3244.

43. Reisz-Porszasz S, Bhasin S, Artaza JN, et al. Lower skeletal muscle mass in male transgenic mice with muscle-specific overexpression of myostatin. *Am J Physiol Endocrinol Metab.* 2003;285(4):E876-E888.

44. Consitt L, Bell J, Houmard J. Intramuscular lipid metabolism, insulin action and obesity. *IUBMB Life.* 2009;61(1):47-55.

45. McCroskery S, Thomas M, Maxwell L, Sharma M, Kambadur R. Myostatin negatively regulates satellite cell activation and self-renewal. *J Cell Biol.* 2003;162(6):1135-1147.

46. Rodin J. Insulin levels, hunger, and food intake: an example of feedback loops in body weight regulation. *Health Psychol.* 1985;4(1):1-24.

47. Kojima M, Hosoda H, Date Y, Nakazato M, Matsuo H, Kangawa K. Ghrelin is a growth-hormone-releasing acylated peptide from stomach. *Nature.* 1999;402(6762):656-660.

48. Wu JT, Kral JG. Ghrelin: integrative neuroendocrine peptide in health and disease. *Ann Surg.* 2004;239(4):464-474.

49. Moller N, Nygren J, Hansen TK, Orskov H, Frystyk J, Nair KS. Splanchnic release of ghrelin in humans. *J Clin Endocrinol Metab.* 2003;88(2):850-852.

50. Ariyasu H, Takaya K, Tagami T, et al. Stomach is a major source of circulating ghrelin, and feeding state determines plasma ghrelin-like immunoreactivity levels in humans. *J Clin Endocrinol Metab.* 2001;86(10):4753-4758.

51. Tassone F, Broglio F, Destefanis S, et al. Neuroendocrine and metabolic effects of acute ghrelin administration in human obesity. *J Clin Endocrinol Metab.* 2003;88(11):5478-5483.

52. Lee HM, Wang G, Englander EW, Kojima M, Greeley GH Jr. Ghrelin, a new gastrointestinal endocrine peptide that stimulates insulin secretion: enteric distribution, ontogeny, influence of endocrine, and dietary manipulations. *Endocrinology.* 2002;143(1):185-190.

53. Toshinai K, Mondal MS, Nakazato M, et al. Upregulation of ghrelin expression in the stomach upon fasting, insulin-induced hypoglycemia, and leptin administration. *Biochem Biophys Res Commun.* 2001;281(5):1220-1225.

54. Hayashida T, Murakami K, Mogi K, et al. Ghrelin in domestic animals: distribution in stomach and its possible role. *Domest Anim Endocrinol.* 2001;21(1):17-24.

55. Qi X, Reed J, Englander EW, Chandrashekar V, Bartke A, Greeley GH Jr. Evidence that growth hormone exerts a feedback effect on stomach ghrelin production and secretion. *Exp Biol Med (Maywood).* 2003;228(9):1028-1032.

56. Broglio F, Arvat E, Benso A, et al. Ghrelin, a natural GH secretagogue produced by the stomach, induces hyperglycemia and reduces insulin secretion in humans. *J Clin Endocrinol Metab.* 2001;86(10):5083-5086.

57. Moesgaard SG, Ahren B, Carr RD, Gram DX, Brand CL, Sundler F. Effects of high-fat feeding and fasting on ghrelin expression in the mouse stomach. *Regul Pept.* 2004;120(1-3):261-267.

58. Sakata I, Tanaka T, Matsubara M, et al. Postnatal changes in ghrelin mRNA expression and in ghrelin-producing cells in the rat stomach. *J Endocrinol.* 2002;174(3):463-471.

59. Date Y, Kojima M, Hosoda H, et al. Ghrelin, a novel growth hormone-releasing acylated peptide, is synthesized in a distinct endocrine cell type in the gastrointestinal tracts of rats and humans. *Endocrinology.* 2000;141(11):4255-4261.

60. Asakawa A, Inui A, Kaga T, et al. Ghrelin is an appetite-stimulatory signal from stomach with structural resemblance to motilin. *Gastroenterology.* 2001;120(2):337-345.

61. Murakami N, Hayashida T, Kuroiwa T, et al. Role for central ghrelin in food intake and secretion profile of stomach ghrelin in rats. *J Endocrinol.* 2002;174(2):283-238.

62. Wren AM, Seal LJ, Cohen MA, et al. Ghrelin enhances appetite and increases food intake in humans. *J Clin Endocrinol Metab.* 2001;86(12):5992.
63. Takaya K, Ariyasu H, Kanamoto N, et al. Ghrelin strongly stimulates growth hormone release in humans. *J Clin Endocrinol Metab.* 2000;85(12):4908-4911.
64. Groschl M, Knerr I, Topf HG, Schmid P, Rascher W, Rauh M. Endocrine responses to the oral ingestion of a physiological dose of essential amino acids in humans. *J Endocrinol.* 2003;179(2):237-244.
65. Enomoto M, Nagaya N, Uematsu M, et al. Cardiovascular and hormonal effects of subcutaneous administration of ghrelin, a novel growth hormone-releasing peptide, in healthy humans. *Clin Sci (Lond).* 2003;105(4):431-435.
66. Broglio F, Benso A, Gottero C, et al. Effects of glucose, free fatty acids or arginine load on the GH-releasing activity of ghrelin in humans. *Clin Endocrinol (Oxf).* 2002;57(2):265-271.
67. Muller AF, Lamberts SW, Janssen JA, et al. Ghrelin drives GH secretion during fasting in man. *Eur J Endocrinol.* 2002;146(2):203-207.
68. Nagaya N, Uematsu M, Kojima M, et al. Elevated circulating level of ghrelin in cachexia associated with chronic heart failure: relationships between ghrelin and anabolic/catabolic factors. *Circulation.* 2001;104(17):2034-2038.
69. Hataya Y, Akamizu T, Takaya K, et al. A low dose of ghrelin stimulates growth hormone (GH) release synergistically with GH-releasing hormone in humans. *J Clin Endocrinol Metab.* 2001;86(9):4552.
70. Peino R, Baldelli R, Rodriguez-Garcia J, et al. Ghrelin-induced growth hormone secretion in humans. *Eur J Endocrinol.* 2000;143(6):R11-R14.
71. Arvat E, Di Vito L, Broglio F, et al. Preliminary evidence that Ghrelin, the natural GH secretagogue (GHS)-receptor ligand, strongly stimulates GH secretion in humans. *J Endocrinol Invest.* 2000;23(8):493-495.
72. Torsello A, Bresciani E, Avallone R, Locatelli V. [Ghrelin and GH secretion.] *Minerva Endocrinol.* 2002;27(4):257-264.
73. Flanagan DE, Evans ML, Monsod TP, et al. The influence of insulin on circulating ghrelin. *Am J Physiol Endocrinol Metab.* 2003;284(2):E313-E316.
74. Monteleone P, Martiadis V, Fabrazzo M, Serritella C, Maj M. Ghrelin and leptin responses to food ingestion in bulimia nervosa: implications for binge-eating and compensatory behaviours. *Psychol Med.* 2003;33(8):1387-1394.
75. Murdolo G, Lucidi P, Di Loreto C, et al. Insulin is required for prandial ghrelin suppression in humans. *Diabetes.* 2003;52(12):2923-2927.
76. Monteleone P, Bencivenga R, Longobardi N, Serritella C, Maj M. Differential responses of circulating ghrelin to high-fat or high-carbohydrate meal in healthy women. *J Clin Endocrinol Metab.* 2003;88(11):5510-5514.
77. Knerr I, Groschl M, Rascher W, Rauh M. Endocrine effects of food intake: insulin, ghrelin, and leptin responses to a single bolus of essential amino acids in humans. *Ann Nutr Metab.* 2003;47(6):312-318.
78. Anderwald C, Brabant G, Bernroider E, et al. Insulin-dependent modulation of plasma ghrelin and leptin concentrations is less pronounced in type 2 diabetic patients. *Diabetes.* 2003;52(7):1792-1798.
79. Nedvidkova J, Krykorkova I, Bartak V, et al. Loss of meal-induced decrease in plasma ghrelin levels in patients with anorexia nervosa. *J Clin Endocrinol Metab.* 2003;88(4):1678-1682.
80. English PJ, Ghatei MA, Malik IA, Bloom SR, Wilding JP. Food fails to suppress ghrelin levels in obese humans. *J Clin Endocrinol Metab.* 2002;87(6):2984.

81. Greenman Y, Golani N, Gilad S, Yaron M, Limor R, Stern N. Ghrelin secretion is modulated in a nutrient- and gender-specific manner. *Clin Endocrinol (Oxf)*. 2004;60(3):382-388.
82. Callahan HS, Cummings DE, Pepe MS, Breen PA, Matthys CC, Weigle DS. Postprandial suppression of plasma ghrelin level is proportional to ingested caloric load but does not predict intermeal interval in humans. *J Clin Endocrinol Metab*. 2004;89(3):1319-1324.
83. Heath RB, Jones R, Frayn KN, Robertson MD. Vagal stimulation exaggerates the inhibitory ghrelin response to oral fat in humans. *J Endocrinol*. 2004;180(2):273-281.
84. Purnell JQ, Weigle DS, Breen P, Cummings DE. Ghrelin levels correlate with insulin levels, insulin resistance, and high-density lipoprotein cholesterol, but not with gender, menopausal status, or cortisol levels in humans. *J Clin Endocrinol Metab*. 2003;88(12):5747-5752.
85. Briatore L, Andraghetti G, Cordera R. Acute plasma glucose increase, but not early insulin response, regulates plasma ghrelin. *Eur J Endocrinol*. 2003;149(5):403-406.
86. Lucidi P, Murdolo G, Di Loreto C, et al. Ghrelin is not necessary for adequate hormonal counterregulation of insulin-induced hypoglycemia. *Diabetes*. 2002;51(10):2911-2914.
87. Caixas A, Bashore C, Nash W, Pi-Sunyer F, Laferrere B. Insulin, unlike food intake, does not suppress ghrelin in human subjects. *J Clin Endocrinol Metab*. 2002;87(4):1902.
88. Marzullo P, Verti B, Savia G, et al. The relationship between active ghrelin levels and human obesity involves alterations in resting energy expenditure. *J Clin Endocrinol Metab*. 2004;89(2):936-939.
89. Soriano-Guillen L, Barrios V, Campos-Barros A, Argente J. Ghrelin levels in obesity and anorexia nervosa: effect of weight reduction or recuperation. *J Pediatr*. 2004;144(1):36-42.
90. Chan JL, Bullen J, Lee JH, Yiannakouris N, Mantzoros CS. Ghrelin levels are not regulated by recombinant leptin administration and/or three days of fasting in healthy subjects. *J Clin Endocrinol Metab*. 2004;89(1):335-343.
91. Malik IA, English PJ, Ghatei MA, Bloom SR, MacFarlane IA, Wilding JP. The relationship of ghrelin to biochemical and anthropometric markers of adult growth hormone deficiency. *Clin Endocrinol (Oxf)*. 2004;60(1):137-141.
92. Krsek M, Rosicka M, Papezova H, et al. Plasma ghrelin levels and malnutrition: a comparison of two etiologies. *Eat Weight Disord*. 2003;8(3):207-211.
93. Fagerberg B, Hulten LM, Hulthe J. Plasma ghrelin, body fat, insulin resistance, and smoking in clinically healthy men: the atherosclerosis and insulin resistance study. *Metabolism*. 2003;52(11):1460-1463.
94. Rosicka M, Krsek M, Matoulek M, et al. Serum ghrelin levels in obese patients: the relationship to serum leptin levels and soluble leptin receptors levels. *Physiol Res*. 2003;52(1):61-66.
95. Lindeman JH, Pijl H, Van Dielen FM, Lentjes EG, Van Leuven C, Kooistra T. Ghrelin and the hyposomatotropism of obesity. *Obes Res*. 2002;10(11):1161-1166.
96. Rigamonti AE, Pincelli AI, Corra B, et al. Plasma ghrelin concentrations in elderly subjects: comparison with anorexic and obese patients. *J Endocrinol*. 2002;175(1):R1-R5.
97. Tanaka M, Naruo T, Muranaga T, et al. Increased fasting plasma ghrelin levels in patients with bulimia nervosa. *Eur J Endocrinol*. 2002;146(6):R1-R3.
98. Bellone S, Rapa A, Vivenza D, et al. Circulating ghrelin levels as function of gender, pubertal status and adiposity in childhood. *J Endocrinol Invest*. 2002;25(5): RC13-RC15.

99. Cummings DE, Weigle DS, Frayo RS, et al. Plasma ghrelin levels after diet-induced weight loss or gastric bypass surgery. *N Engl J Med.* 2002;346(21):1623-1630.
100. Hansen TK, Dall R, Hosoda H, et al. Weight loss increases circulating levels of ghrelin in human obesity. *Clin Endocrinol (Oxf).* 2002;56(2):203-206.
101. Otto B, Cuntz U, Fruehauf E, et al. Weight gain decreases elevated plasma ghrelin concentrations of patients with anorexia nervosa. *Eur J Endocrinol.* 2001;145(5): 669-673.
102. Tschop M, Weyer C, Tataranni PA, Devanarayan V, Ravussin E, Heiman ML. Circulating ghrelin levels are decreased in human obesity. *Diabetes.* 2001;50(4): 707-709.
103. Barkan AL, Dimaraki EV, Jessup SK, Symons KV, Ermolenko M, Jaffe CA. Ghrelin secretion in humans is sexually dimorphic, suppressed by somatostatin, and not affected by the ambient growth hormone levels. *J Clin Endocrinol Metab.* 2003;88(5):2180-2184.
104. Gaytan F, Barreiro ML, Caminos JE, et al. Expression of ghrelin and its functional receptor, the type 1a growth hormone secretagogue receptor, in normal human testis and testicular tumors. *J Clin Endocrinol Metab.* 2004;89(1):400-409.
105. Pagotto U, Gambineri A, Pelusi C, et al. Testosterone replacement therapy restores normal ghrelin in hypogonadal men. *J Clin Endocrinol Metab.* 2003;88(9):4139-4143.
106. Pagotto U, Gambineri A, Vicennati V, Heiman ML, Tschop M, Pasquali R. Plasma ghrelin, obesity, and the polycystic ovary syndrome: correlation with insulin resistance and androgen levels. *J Clin Endocrinol Metab.* 2002;87(12):5625-5629.
107. Miraglia del Giudice E, Santoro N, Cirillo G, et al. Molecular screening of the ghrelin gene in Italian obese children: the Leu72Met variant is associated with an earlier onset of obesity. *Int J Obes Relat Metab Disord.* 2004;28(3):447-450.
108. Neary NM, Small CJ, Bloom SR. Gut and mind. *Gut.* 2003;52(7):918-921.
109. Zigman JM, Elmquist JK. Minireview: from anorexia to obesity–the yin and yang of body weight control. *Endocrinology.* 2003;144(9):3749-3756.
110. Holdstock C, Engstrom BE, Ohrvall M, Lind L, Sundbom M, Karlsson FA. Ghrelin and adipose tissue regulatory peptides: effect of gastric bypass surgery in obese humans. *J Clin Endocrinol Metab.* 2003;88(7):3177-3183.
111. Murdolo G, Lucidi P, Di Loreto C, et al. Circulating ghrelin levels of visceral obese men are not modified by a short-term treatment with very low doses of GH replacement. *J Endocrinol Invest.* 2003;26(3):244-249.
112. Tritos NA, Kokkinos A, Lampadariou E, Alexiou E, Katsilambros N, Maratos-Flier E. Cerebrospinal fluid ghrelin is negatively associated with body mass index. *J Clin Endocrinol Metab.* 2003;88(6):2943-2946.
113. Shiiya T, Nakazato M, Mizuta M, et al. Plasma ghrelin levels in lean and obese humans and the effect of glucose on ghrelin secretion. *J Clin Endocrinol Metab.* 2002;87(1):240-244.
114. Popovic V, Miljic D, Micic D, et al. Ghrelin main action on the regulation of growth hormone release is exerted at hypothalamic level. *J Clin Endocrinol Metab.* 2003;88(7):3450-3453.
115. Arosio M, Ronchi CL, Gebbia C, Cappiello V, Beck-Peccoz P, Peracchi M. Stimulatory effects of ghrelin on circulating somatostatin and pancreatic polypeptide levels. *J Clin Endocrinol Metab.* 2003;88(2):701-704.
116. Tschop M, Wawarta R, Riepl RL, et al. Post-prandial decrease of circulating human ghrelin levels. *J Endocrinol Invest.* 2001;24(6):RC19-RC21.
117. Inui A, Asakawa A, Bowers CY, et al. Ghrelin, appetite, and gastric motility: the emerging role of the stomach as an endocrine organ. *FASEB J.* 2004;18(3):439-456.

118. Cummings DE, Purnell JQ, Frayo RS, Schmidova K, Wisse BE, Weigle DS. A pre-prandial rise in plasma ghrelin levels suggests a role in meal initiation in humans. *Diabetes.* 2001;50(8):1714-1719.
119. Weikel JC, Wichniak A, Ising M, et al. Ghrelin promotes slow-wave sleep in humans. *Am J Physiol Endocrinol Metab.* 2003;284(2):E407-E415.
120. Tritos NA, Mun E, Bertkau A, Grayson R, Maratos-Flier E, Goldfine A. Serum ghrelin levels in response to glucose load in obese subjects post-gastric bypass surgery. *Obes Res.* 2003;11(8):919-924.
121. Pelleymounter MA, Cullen MJ, Baker MB, et al. Effects of the obese gene product on body weight regulation in ob/ob mice. *Science.* 1995;269(5223):540-543.
122. Halaas JL, Gajiwala KS, Maffei M, et al. Weight-reducing effects of the plasma protein encoded by the obese gene. *Science.* 1995;269(5223):543-546.
123. Campfield LA, Smith FJ, Guisez Y, Devos R, Burn P. Recombinant mouse OB protein: evidence for a peripheral signal linking adiposity and central neural networks. *Science.* 1995;269(5223):546-549.
124. Montague CT, Farooqi IS, Whitehead JP, et al. Congenital leptin deficiency is associated with severe early-onset obesity in humans. *Nature.* 1997;387(6636):903-908.
125. Clement K, Vaisse C, Lahlou N, et al. A mutation in the human leptin receptor gene causes obesity and pituitary dysfunction. *Nature.* 1998;392(6674):398-401.
126. Carlsson B, Lindell K, Gabrielsson B, et al. Obese (ob) gene defects are rare in human obesity. *Obes Res.* 1997;5(1):30-35.
127. Campfield LA, Smith FJ, Burn P. The OB protein (leptin) pathway–a link between adipose tissue mass and central neural networks. *Horm Metab Res.* 1996;28(12):619-632.
128. Moinat M, Deng C, Muzzin P, et al. Modulation of obese gene expression in rat brown and white adipose tissues. *FEBS Lett.* 1995;373(2):131-134.
129. Klein S, Coppack SW, Mohamed-Ali V, Landt M. Adipose tissue leptin production and plasma leptin kinetics in humans. *Diabetes.* 1996;45(7):984-987.
130. Ronnemaa T, Karonen SL, Rissanen A, Koskenvuo M, Koivisto VA. Relation between plasma leptin levels and measures of body fat in identical twins discordant for obesity. *Ann Intern Med.* 1997;126(1):26-31.
131. Lonnqvist F, Nordfors L, Jansson M, Thorne A, Schalling M, Arner P. Leptin secretion from adipose tissue in women. Relationship to plasma levels and gene expression. *J Clin Invest.* 1997;99(10):2398-2404.
132. Minocci A, Savia G, Lucantoni R, et al. Leptin plasma concentrations are dependent on body fat distribution in obese patients. *Int J Obes Relat Metab Disord.* 2000;24(9):1139-1144.
133. Considine RV, Sinha MK, Heiman ML, et al. Serum immunoreactive-leptin concentrations in normal-weight and obese humans. *N Engl J Med.* 1996;334(5):292-295.
134. Shimizu H, Shimomura Y, Hayashi R, et al. Serum leptin concentration is associated with total body fat mass, but not abdominal fat distribution. *Int J Obes Relat Metab Disord.* 1997;21(7):536-541.
135. Fisher JS, Hickner RC, Racette SB, Binder EF, Landt M, Kohrt WM. Leptin response to insulin in humans is related to the lipolytic state of abdominal subcutaneous fat. *J Clin Endocrinol Metab.* 1999;84(10):3726-3731.
136. Van Harmelen V, Reynisdottir S, Eriksson P, et al. Leptin secretion from subcutaneous and visceral adipose tissue in women. *Diabetes.* 1998;47(6):913-917.
137. Hube F, Lietz U, Igel M, et al. Difference in leptin mRNA levels between omental and subcutaneous abdominal adipose tissue from obese humans. *Horm Metab Res.* 1996;28(12):690-693.

138. Taylor RW, Goulding A. Plasma leptin in relation to regional body fat in older New Zealand women. *Aust N Z J Med.* 1998;28(3):316-321.
139. Ostlund RE Jr, Yang JW, Klein S, Gingerich R. Relation between plasma leptin concentration and body fat, gender, diet, age, and metabolic covariates. *J Clin Endocrinol Metab.* 1996;81(11):3909-3913.
140. Hickey MS, Considine RV, Israel RG, et al. Leptin is related to body fat content in male distance runners. *Am J Physiol.* 1996;271(5 Pt 1):E938-E940.
141. Wauters M, Mertens I, Considine R, De Leeuw I, Van Gaal L. Are leptin levels dependent on body fat distribution in obese men and women? *Eat Weight Disord.* 1998;3(3):124-130.
142. Hassink SG, Sheslow DV, de Lancey E, Opentanova I, Considine RV, Caro JF. Serum leptin in children with obesity: relationship to gender and development. *Pediatrics.* 1996;98(2 Pt 1):201-203.
143. Moller N, O'Brien P, Nair KS. Disruption of the relationship between fat content and leptin levels with aging in humans. *J Clin Endocrinol Metab.* 1998;83(3):931-934.
144. Ranganathan S, Maffei M, Kern PA. Adipose tissue ob mRNA expression in humans: discordance with plasma leptin and relationship with adipose TNFalpha expression. *J Lipid Res.* 1998;39(4):724-730.
145. Garcia-Lorda P, Bullo M, Vila R, del Mar Grasa M, Alemany M, Salas-Salvado J. Leptin concentrations do not correlate with fat mass nor with metabolic risk factors in morbidly obese females. *Diabetes Nutr Metab.* 2001;14(6):329-336.
146. Johannsson G, Karlsson C, Lonn L, et al. Serum leptin concentration and insulin sensitivity in men with abdominal obesity. *Obes Res.* 1998;6(6):416-421.
147. Cnop M, Landchild MJ, Vidal J, et al. The concurrent accumulation of intra-abdominal and subcutaneous fat explains the association between insulin resistance and plasma leptin concentrations: distinct metabolic effects of two fat compartments. *Diabetes.* 2002;51(4):1005-1015.
148. Takahashi M, Funahashi T, Shimomura I, Miyaoka K, Matsuzawa Y. Plasma leptin levels and body fat distribution. *Horm Metab Res.* 1996;28(12):751-752.
149. Montague CT, Prins JB, Sanders L, Digby JE, O'Rahilly S. Depot- and sex-specific differences in human leptin mRNA expression: implications for the control of regional fat distribution. *Diabetes.* 1997;46(3):342-347.
150. Elias CF, Lee C, Kelly J, et al. Leptin activates hypothalamic CART neurons projecting to the spinal cord. *Neuron.* 1998;21(6):1375-1385.
151. Morley JE, Alshaher MM, Farr SA, Flood JF, Kumar VB. Leptin and neuropeptide Y (NPY) modulate nitric oxide synthase: further evidence for a role of nitric oxide in feeding. *Peptides.* 1999;20(5):595-600.
152. Barba G, Russo O, Siani A, et al. Plasma leptin and blood pressure in men: graded association independent of body mass and fat pattern. *Obes Res.* 2003;11(1):160-166.
153. Mistry AM, Swick AG, Romsos DR. Leptin rapidly lowers food intake and elevates metabolic rates in lean and ob/ob mice. *J Nutr.* 1997;127(10):2065-2072.
154. William WN Jr, Ceddia RB, Curi R. Leptin controls the fate of fatty acids in isolated rat white adipocytes. *J Endocrinol.* 2002;175(3):735-744.
155. Fruhbeck G, Gomez-Ambrosi J. Depot-specific differences in the lipolytic effect of leptin on isolated white adipocytes. *Med Sci Monit.* 2002;8(2):BR47-BR55.
156. Fruhbeck G, Gomez-Ambrosi J, Salvador J. Leptin-induced lipolysis opposes the tonic inhibition of endogenous adenosine in white adipocytes. *FASEB J.* 2001;15(2):333-340.
157. Fruhbeck G, Aguado M, Martinez JA. In vitro lipolytic effect of leptin on mouse adipocytes: evidence for a possible autocrine/paracrine role of leptin. *Biochem Biophys Res Commun.* 1997;240(3):590-594.

158. Kamohara S, Burcelin R, Halaas JL, Friedman JM, Charron MJ. Acute stimulation of glucose metabolism in mice by leptin treatment. *Nature.* 1997;389(6649):374-377.

159. Ramsay TG. Porcine leptin alters insulin inhibition of lipolysis in porcine adipocytes in vitro. *J Anim Sci.* 2001;79(3):653-657.

160. Wang MY, Lee Y, Unger RH. Novel form of lipolysis induced by leptin. *J Biol Chem.* 1999;274(25):17541-17544.

161. Siegrist-Kaiser CA, Pauli V, Juge-Aubry CE, et al. Direct effects of leptin on brown and white adipose tissue. *J Clin Invest.* 1997;100(11):2858-2864.

162. Fruhbeck G, Aguado M, Gomez-Ambrosi J, Martinez JA. Lipolytic effect of in vivo leptin administration on adipocytes of lean and ob/ob mice, but not db/db mice. *Biochem Biophys Res Commun.* 1998;250(1):99-102.

163. Wang ZW, Zhou YT, Lee Y, Higa M, Kalra SP, Unger RH. Hyperleptinemia depletes fat from denervated fat tissue. *Biochem Biophys Res Commun.* 1999;260(3):653-657.

164. Ramsay TG. Porcine leptin inhibits lipogenesis in porcine adipocytes. *J Anim Sci.* 2003;81(12):3008-3017.

165. Ceddia RB, William WN Jr, Lima FB, Flandin P, Curi R, Giacobino JP. Leptin stimulates uncoupling protein-2 mRNA expression and Krebs cycle activity and inhibits lipid synthesis in isolated rat white adipocytes. *Eur J Biochem.* 2000;267(19):5952-5958.

166. Ceddia RB, William WN Jr, Lima FB, Curi R. Leptin inhibits insulin-stimulated incorporation of glucose into lipids and stimulates glucose decarboxylation in isolated rat adipocytes. *J Endocrinol.* 1998;158(3):R7-R9.

167. Elimam A, Kamel A, Marcus C. In vitro effects of leptin on human adipocyte metabolism. *Horm Res.* 2002;58(2):88-93.

168. Zhang HH, Kumar S, Barnett AH, Eggo MC. Intrinsic site-specific differences in the expression of leptin in human adipocytes and its autocrine effects on glucose uptake. *J Clin Endocrinol Metab.* 1999;84(7):2550-2556.

169. Hellstrom L, Wahrenberg H, Hruska K, Reynisdottir S, Arner P. Mechanisms behind gender differences in circulating leptin levels. *J Intern Med.* 2000;247(4):457-462.

170. Couillard C, Mauriege P, Prud'homme D, et al. Plasma leptin concentrations: gender differences and associations with metabolic risk factors for cardiovascular disease. *Diabetologia.* 1997;40(10):1178-1184.

171. Niskanen LK, Haffner S, Karhunen LJ, Turpeinen AK, Miettinen H, Uusitupa MI. Serum leptin in obesity is related to gender and body fat topography but does not predict successful weight loss. *Eur J Endocrinol.* 1997;137(1):61-67.

172. Vettor R, De Pergola G, Pagano C, et al. Gender differences in serum leptin in obese people: relationships with testosterone, body fat distribution and insulin sensitivity. *Eur J Clin Invest.* 1997;27(12):1016-1024.

173. Jensen MD, Hensrud D, O'Brien PC, Nielsen S. Collection and interpretation of plasma leptin concentration data in humans. *Obes Res.* 1999;7(3):241-245.

174. Di Marzo V, Goparaju SK, Wang L, et al. Leptin-regulated endocannabinoids are involved in maintaining food intake. *Nature.* 2001;410(6830):822-825.

175. Baskin DG, Seeley RJ, Kuijper JL, et al. Increased expression of mRNA for the long form of the leptin receptor in the hypothalamus is associated with leptin hypersensitivity and fasting. *Diabetes.* 1998;47(4):538-543.

176. Backberg M, Hervieu G, Wilson S, Meister B. Orexin receptor-1 (OX-R1) immunoreactivity in chemically identified neurons of the hypothalamus: focus on orexin targets involved in control of food and water intake. *Eur J Neurosci.* 2002;15(2):315-328.

177. Sahu A. Evidence suggesting that galanin (GAL), melanin-concentrating hormone (MCH), neurotensin (NT), proopiomelanocortin (POMC) and neuropeptide Y (NPY) are targets of leptin signaling in the hypothalamus. *Endocrinology.* 1998;139(2):795-798.

178. Kristensen P, Judge ME, Thim L, et al. Hypothalamic CART is a new anorectic peptide regulated by leptin. *Nature.* 1998;393(6680):72-76.

179. Baskin DG, Breininger JF, Schwartz MW. Leptin receptor mRNA identifies a subpopulation of neuropeptide Y neurons activated by fasting in rat hypothalamus. *Diabetes.* 1999;48(4):828-833.

180. Mercer JG, Moar KM, Rayner DV, Trayhurn P, Hoggard N. Regulation of leptin receptor and NPY gene expression in hypothalamus of leptin-treated obese (ob/ob) and cold-exposed lean mice. *FEBS Lett.* 1997;402(2-3):185-188.

181. Schwartz MW, Baskin DG, Bukowski TR, et al. Specificity of leptin action on elevated blood glucose levels and hypothalamic neuropeptide Y gene expression in ob/ob mice. *Diabetes.* 1996;45(4):531-535.

182. Elmquist JK. Hypothalamic pathways underlying the endocrine, autonomic, and behavioral effects of leptin. *Physiol Behav.* 2001;74(4-5):703-708.

183. Stephens TW, Basinski M, Bristow PK, et al. The role of neuropeptide Y in the anti-obesity action of the obese gene product. *Nature.* 1995;377(6549):530-532.

184. Mercer JG, Hoggard N, Williams LM, et al. Coexpression of leptin receptor and preproneuropeptide Y mRNA in arcuate nucleus of mouse hypothalamus. *J Neuroendocrinol.* 1996;8(10):733-735.

185. Cheung CC, Clifton DK, Steiner RA. Proopiomelanocortin neurons are direct targets for leptin in the hypothalamus. *Endocrinology.* 1997;138(10):4489-4492.

186. Schwartz MW, Seeley RJ, Campfield LA, Burn P, Baskin DG. Identification of targets of leptin action in rat hypothalamus. *J Clin Invest.* 1996;98(5):1101-1106.

187. Shimada M, Tritos NA, Lowell BB, Flier JS, Maratos-Flier E. Mice lacking melanin-concentrating hormone are hypophagic and lean. *Nature.* 1998;396(6712):670-674.

188. Proulx K, Richard D, Walker CD. Leptin regulates appetite-related neuropeptides in the hypothalamus of developing rats without affecting food intake. *Endocrinology.* 2002;143(12):4683-4692.

189. Hosoi T, Okuma Y, Nomura Y. Leptin regulates interleukin-1beta expression in the brain via the STAT3-independent mechanisms. *Brain Res.* 2002;949(1-2):139-146.

190. Korner J, Savontaus E, Chua SC Jr, Leibel RL, Wardlaw SL. Leptin regulation of Agrp and Npy mRNA in the rat hypothalamus. *J Neuroendocrinol.* 2001;13(11):959-966.

191. Niimi M, Sato M, Taminato T. Neuropeptide Y in central control of feeding and interactions with orexin and leptin. *Endocrine.* 2001;14(2):269-273.

192. Schwartz MW, Erickson JC, Baskin DG, Palmiter RD. Effect of fasting and leptin deficiency on hypothalamic neuropeptide Y gene transcription in vivo revealed by expression of a lacZ reporter gene. *Endocrinology.* 1998;139(5):2629-2635.

193. Hosoi T, Okuma Y, Nomura Y. Leptin induces IL-1 receptor antagonist expression in the brain. *Biochem Biophys Res Commun.* 2002;294(2):215-219.

194. Funahashi H, Hori T, Shimoda Y, et al. Morphological evidence for neural interactions between leptin and orexin in the hypothalamus. *Regul Pept.* 2000;92(1-3):31-35.

195. Goldstone AP, Mercer JG, Gunn I, et al. Leptin interacts with glucagon-like peptide-1 neurons to reduce food intake and body weight in rodents. *FEBS Lett.* 1997;415(2):134-138.

196. Dryden S, King P, Pickavance L, Doyle P, Williams G. Divergent effects of intracerebroventricular and peripheral leptin administration on feeding and hypothalamic neuropeptide Y in lean and obese (fa/fa) Zucker rats. *Clin Sci (Lond).* 1999;96(3):307-312.

197. Cohen P, Zhao C, Cai X, et al. Selective deletion of leptin receptor in neurons leads to obesity. *J Clin Invest.* 2001;108(8):1113-1121.

198. Pinto S, Roseberry AG, Liu H, et al. Rapid rewiring of arcuate nucleus feeding circuits by leptin. *Science.* 2004;304(5667):110-115.

199. Brunner L, Nick HP, Cumin F, et al. Leptin is a physiologically important regulator of food intake. *Int J Obes Relat Metab Disord*. 1997;21(12):1152-1160.
200. Rentsch J, Levens N, Chiesi M. Recombinant ob-gene product reduces food intake in fasted mice. *Biochem Biophys Res Commun*. 1995;214(1):131-136.
201. Rosenbaum M, Nicolson M, Hirsch J, et al. Effects of gender, body composition, and menopause on plasma concentrations of leptin. *J Clin Endocrinol Metab*. 1996;81(9):3424-3427.
202. Giovambattista A, Suescun MO, Nessralla CC, Franca LR, Spinedi E, Calandra RS. Modulatory effects of leptin on leydig cell function of normal and hyperleptinemic rats. *Neuroendocrinology*. 2003;78(5):270-279.
203. Sun C, Yu C, Wang S. Study on the effects of leptin on puberty development in children. *Zhonghua Yu Fang Yi Xue Za Zhi*. 2001;35(5):293-296.
204. Mounzih K, Lu R, Chehab FF. Leptin treatment rescues the sterility of genetically obese ob/ob males. *Endocrinology*. 1997;138(3):1190-1193.
205. Pralong FP, Gonzales C, Voirol MJ, et al. The neuropeptide Y Y1 receptor regulates leptin-mediated control of energy homeostasis and reproductive functions. *FASEB J*. 2002;16(7):712-714.
206. Barash IA, Cheung CC, Weigle DS, et al. Leptin is a metabolic signal to the reproductive system. *Endocrinology*. 1996;137:3144-3147.
207. Chehab FF, Lim ME, Lu R. Correction of the sterility defect homozygous obese female mice by treatment with the human recombinant leptin. *Nat Genet*. 1996;12:318-320.
208. Strobel A, Issad T, Camoin L, Ozata M, Strosberg AD. A leptin missense mutation associated with hypogonadism and morbid obesity. *Nat Genet*. 1998;139:2284-2286.
209. Tezuka M, Irahara M, Ogura K, et al. Effects of leptin on gonadotropin secretion in juvenile female rat pituitary cells. *Eur J Endocrinol*. 2002;146(2):261-266.
210. Kiess W, Reich A, Meyer K, et al. A role for leptin in sexual maturation and puberty? *Horm Res*. 1999;51(Suppl 3):55-63.
211. Ellis KJ, Nicolson M. Leptin levels and body fatness in children: effects of gender, ethnicity, and sexual development. *Pediatr Res*. 1997;42(4):484-488.
212. Gueorguiev M, Goth ML, Korbonits M. Leptin and puberty: a review. *Pituitary*. 2001;4(1-2):79-86.
213. Ahima RS, Dushay J, Flier SN, Prabakaran D, Flier JS. Leptin accelerates the onset of puberty in normal female mice. *J Clin Invest*. 1997;99(3):391-395.
214. Yura S, Ogawa Y, Sagawa N, et al. Accelerated puberty and late-onset hypothalamic hypogonadism in female transgenic skinny mice overexpressing leptin. *J Clin Invest*. 2000;105(6):749-755.
215. Bronson FH. Puberty in female mice is not associated with increases in either body fat or leptin. *Endocrinology*. 2001;142(11):4758-4761.
216. Chehab FF, Mounzih K, Lu R, Lim ME. Early onset of reproductive function in normal female mice treated with leptin. *Science*. 1997;275(5296):88-90.
217. Cheung CC, Thornton JE, Kuijper JL, Weigle DS, Clifton DK, Steiner RA. Leptin is a metabolic gate for the onset of puberty in the female rat. *Endocrinology*. 1997;138(2):855-858.
218. Cheung CC, Thornton JE, Nurani SD, Clifton DK, Steiner RA. A reassessment of leptin's role in triggering the onset of puberty in the rat and mouse. *Neuroendocrinology*. 2001;74(1):12-21.
219. Mantzoros CS, Flier JS, Rogol AD. A longitudinal assessment of hormonal and physical alterations during normal puberty in boys. V. Rising leptin levels may signal the onset of puberty. *J Clin Endocrinol Metab*. 1997;82(4):1066-1070.

220. Gruaz NM, Lalaoui M, Pierroz DD, et al. Chronic administration of leptin into the lateral ventricle induces sexual maturation in severely food-restricted female rats. *J Neuroendocrinol.* 1998;10(8):627-633.
221. Brandao CM, Lombardi MT, Nishida SK, Hauache OM, Vieira JG. Serum leptin concentration during puberty in healthy nonobese adolescents. *Braz J Med Biol Res.* 2003;36(10):1293-1296.
222. Weimann E, Blum WF, Witzel C, Schwidergall S, Bohles HJ. Hypoleptinemia in female and male elite gymnasts. *Eur J Clin Invest.* 1999;29(10):853-860.
223. Shigemura N, Ohta R, Kusakabe Y, et al. Leptin modulates behavioral responses to sweet substances by influencing peripheral taste structures. *Endocrinology.* 2004;145(2):839-847.
224. Blum WF, Englaro P, Hanitsch S, et al. Plasma leptin levels in healthy children and adolescents: dependence on body mass index, body fat mass, gender, pubertal stage, and testosterone. *J Clin Endocrinol Metab.* 1997;82(9):2904-2910.
225. Samra JS, Clark ML, Humphreys SM, et al. Effects of morning rise in cortisol concentration on regulation of lipolysis in subcutaneous adipose tissue. *Am J Physiol.* 1996;271(6 Pt 1):E996-1002.
226. Born J, Kern W, Bieber K, et al. Night-time plasma cortisol secretion is associated with specific sleep stages. *Biol Psychiatry.* 1986;21(14):1415-1424.
227. Kawai K, Sugimoto K, Nakashima K, Miura H, Ninomiya Y. Leptin as a modulator of sweet taste sensitivities in mice. *Proc Natl Acad Sci U S A.* 2000;97(20):11044-11049.
228. Shigemura N, Miura H, Kusakabe Y, Hino A, Ninomiya Y. Expression of leptin receptor (Ob-R) isoforms and signal transducers and activators of transcription (STATs) mRNAs in the mouse taste buds. *Arch Histol Cytol.* 2003;66(3):253-260.
229. Han Z, Yan JQ, Luo GG, Liu Y, Wang YL. Leptin receptor expression in the basolateral nucleus of amygdala of conditioned taste aversion rats. *World J Gastroenterol.* 2003;9(5):1034-1037.
230. Martin-Romero C, Santos-Alvarez J, Goberna R, Sanchez-Margalet V. Human leptin enhances activation and proliferation of human circulating T lymphocytes. *Cell Immunol.* 2000;199(1):15-24.
231. Lord GM, Matarese G, Howard JK, Baker RJ, Bloom SR, Lechler RI. Leptin modulates the T-cell immune response and reverses starvation-induced immunosuppression. *Nature.* 1998;394(6696):897-901.
232. Sasai K, Oba K, Nakano H, Metori S. [Effect of age, gender, and body fat distribution on serum leptin concentrations]. *Nippon Ronen Igakkai Zasshi.* 1999;36(12):874-880.
233. Scarpace PJ, Tumer N. Peripheral and hypothalamic leptin resistance with age-related obesity. *Physiol Behav.* 2001;74(4-5):721-727.
234. Muzzin P, Eisensmith RC, Copeland KC, Woo SL. Correction of obesity and diabetes in genetically obese mice by leptin gene therapy. *Proc Natl Acad Sci U S A.* 1996;93(25):14804-14808.
235. Meister B. Control of food intake via leptin receptors in the hypothalamus. *Vitam Horm.* 2000;59:265-304.
236. Heini AF, Lara-Castro C, Kirk KA, Considine RV, Caro JF, Weinsier RL. Association of leptin and hunger-satiety ratings in obese women. *Int J Obes Relat Metab Disord.* 1998;22(11):1084-1087.
237. Lado-Abeal J, Norman RL. Leptin and reproductive function in males. *Semin Reprod Med.* 2002;20(2):145-151.
238. Bornstein SR, Licinio J, Tauchnitz R, et al. Plasma leptin levels are increased in survivors of acute sepsis: associated loss of diurnal rhythm, in cortisol and leptin secretion. *J Clin Endocrinol Metab.* 1998;83(1):280-283.

It is difficult to write salient points about how to eat if certain assumptions we have about diet are disagreed upon. Many publications still espouse viewpoints that have been long disproven; therefore, this chapter will head off some important misconceptions so that we may think beyond half-truths and full out inaccuracies, and only then can we build a foundation of diet in order to help athletes reach their goals.

This chapter is a compilation of the most common and important myths about nutrition, including communal questions such as, "Is a calorie a calorie?"; "Is there a perfect diet?"; and "Is red meat bad for you?" There will also be information on cholesterol and its role in heart disease, eating small frequent meals as opposed to fewer and larger ones, how protein consumption affects your kidneys, whether being gluten-free or vegan is healthy or necessary, and how beneficial (or not) eating organic foods can be.

Knowing where certain myths stem from may give the reader a better idea for why they are, in fact, myths. Some come from poor science and some just from media stories that caught fire and were never opposed, but as innocent as they seem, some of these myths are dangerous and occasionally set our knowledge of nutrition back decades.

Nutrition Myths and Clarifications

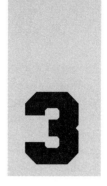

KEY TAKEAWAY

* There are various reasons why certain nutrition myths are so entrenched in culture, such as media stories, poor science, or indifference of the public.

COMMON MYTHS AND WHERE THEY CAME FROM

The Myth: A Calorie Is a Calorie

The body is a complex biological system with intricate processes that regulate energy balance. Different foods go through different biochemical pathways, some of which are inefficient and cause energy to be lost as heat.[1]

The first 2 laws of thermodynamics are seemingly the most relevant to the systems considered in nutrition, or at least the most talked about.

The first law of thermodynamics that says energy is neither created nor destroyed must somehow say that 100 calories of carbohydrates will produce identical effects as the same amount of calories from protein or fat. The problem is that the first law describes a closed system not affected by the outside environment, so the human body is not a great example as we are all affected one way or another by the environment surrounding us easily changing how the inside of our bodies operate. It does state that the total energy of the system before and after must be the same, so it does apply; however, it says nothing about the efficiency or inefficiency of the body in

Amato D. *An Athletic Trainer's Guide to Sports Nutrition (pp 31-42).*

converting that food to energy. Since the law gives us no information about efficiency, the first law cannot tell us if eating different macronutrients cause identical reactions. Even more important is the fact that different foods and macronutrients have a major effect on the hormones and brain centers that control hunger and eating behavior.

The second law is what describes efficiency. Efficiency is how much work you can get done based on how much energy is put in, much like your car engine that is roughly 33% efficient, which means that one-third of the energy you put in (the chemical energy stored in the gasoline) does work; the other two-thirds is thrown off as heat.

The body works much the same way. On a government-recommended diet of about 60% carbs, the human body also wastes about two-thirds of the ingested energy as heat. If you add ethanol to gasoline, your fuel economy goes down. If you add hydrocarbons, your efficiency goes up.

This is exactly why we get our ratios for calorie values. Fat is 9 calories/gram, carbs are 4 calories, and protein is 4 calories. Atwater and Woods distinguished between physical fuel values and physiological fuel values.[2] The first, physical fuel values, is the amount of energy you can get out of food by burning it with oxygen, literally. The body may burn fat using one set of enzymes over another—like the difference between aerobic (burning in the presence of oxygen) and anaerobic (burning in the absence of oxygen)—or may upregulate the production of fat burning enzymes to make the whole process more efficient. These 2 require different enzymes and other molecules. Different or accelerated avenues of metabolization can produce different amounts of energy.

The physical and physiological fuel values do not match up for protein either. It takes energy to process the food we eat, energy that is wasted as heat, known as the *thermic effect of food* (TEF). When you eat a meal, you warm up; it is that simple. There is an extensive amount of research on the subject: about 2% of the ingested calories of fat, 7% of carbs, and 30% of protein is wasted as heat whenever you eat.[3]

The Facts

While there are many different diet compositions that can work, not every one will work for every individual. Genetic, lifestyle, and activity level variations are just a few factors that can dictate what may work for a specific person. While conventional wisdom may espouse the narrative that "it doesn't matter as long as you don't eat too many calories," this is an incomplete statement. A **ketogenic diet** (very high fat, very low carb, moderate protein) causes multiple metabolic and cellular changes within the body that are much different than a very low fat, high carb diet. While normalizing for calorie intake may produce similar short-term results, it does not tell us anything about the overall health and long-term effect on an individual. Each athlete is different and needs an individualized plan in order to optimize performance and health.

The Myth: There Is One Perfect Diet

Various populations around the world have different levels of overall health that are caused by countless factors. We can disseminate which information correlates best to certain markers of health like stress, exercise, and diet. There are many populations that have similarly respectable health statuses but eat very differently. This is likely highly factored by genetic predisposition, one of the biggest reasons why there is no perfect diet and each of us should be thought of as an individual.

The Kitavan population in the Pacific Islands thrives with very low levels of cardiovascular disease and metabolic syndrome, and their diet is composed of about 70% white rice and sweet potatoes, a very high carb diet,[4] while inhabitants on the isle of Crete have the lowest mortality rate and incidence of cancer of European nations.[5] The Cretan's diet is composed of about 40% fat, mostly from olive oil. These are just 2 examples of vastly different diet compositions yet similarly healthy populations.

The Facts

There is no perfect diet, but there is a perfect diet at a specific time for a specific goal.[6] What works for some athletes may not by optimal or even recommended for other athletes because differences in gene expression, body fat percentage, activity level and type, and specific goals will determine what makes the most sense.

The Myth: Red Meat Causes Cancer and Heart Disease

Every now and then a news story breaks with a headline telling us how red meat will kill you, typically citing a research paper that was not even investigating that specifically, with very weak (if any) correlation. Most notably was a recent study from 2011 that made the claim that processed red meat caused a 17% increase in developing bowel cancer in meat eaters as opposed to non–red meat eaters. That statistic by itself is not very compelling and is even less so when actually crunching the data. The study was done in the United Kingdom, where the incidence of bowel cancer is 61 people per 1000, so for every 1000 people in the UK, 61 of them will develop bowel cancer at some point in their life. The part of the population that ate less processed meat had a relative risk reduction of 17%, not an absolute risk reduction.[7]

The headline and abstract lead us to believe that if one eats less processed red meat, the absolute bowel cancer risk reduction goes down 17%. That is not correct. Since the study showed a relative risk reduction, the bowel cancer rate among people who ate less processed red meat was 51 people per 1000, a 17% relative risk reduction, or a difference of 10 people per 1000—not exactly compelling numbers to show a correlation to bowel cancer.

To put these figures into context, if you have a study population of 100 people and normally 10 of them get X disease and the study shows an intervention produces a risk reduction 20%, the investigators would put that at the forefront of the article. However, reading that in the abstract may seem like a powerful statistic in absolute terms, which means that exactly 2 fewer people got X disease.

The Fact

Though quality of red meat varies depending on source, treatment of the animal, environment, and nutrition of the animal, there is no distinct correlation between incidence of cancer of any kind and consumption of red meat with enough compelling evidence to be reproduced.

The Myth: You Can Out-Train Your Diet

Perhaps one of the biggest misconceptions athletes or the general population have about the "calories in/calories out" equation is that it is just simple math: burn more calories than you eat and you will lose weight. That proclamation has a lot of things wrong with it, however. First, there are many calculators that show how many calories you will expend throughout a 24-hour period based on your height and weight, but this is very misleading. None of these calculations take into account regulation of your thyroid hormone, the hormone mainly responsible for your metabolic rate, nor the amount of lean mass you have (muscle burns calories, but fat tissue does not). There are also genetic and epigenetic differences that account for calorie burn, so making a blanket statement about how many calories you should eat on a daily basis is faulty.

In addition, all calories are not created equal. The TEF is an important part of the equation and must be well understood. Each macronutrient requires a unique amount of energy in order to process it to be used within the body. Carbs require about 5% to 10% of their calories just to be metabolized into energy, churned in the stomach, etc. Fats only require 0% to 3%, and protein takes up about 20% to 30%. The net calorie count of 100 g of protein is therefore not nearly the same as 100 g of fat. We have also seen that it does not take as much energy to digest some processed foods as it does whole foods.[8] In other words, what happens hormonally and metabolically when you ingest 100 calories of watermelon is not the same as 100 calories of beef jerky or a twinkie.

The overriding concept here is that unless you are a professional athlete, it is not likely you will be able to eat anything you want and then try to "exercise it off." That is eloquently explained in a study done comparing energy expenditure while either walking or running. To simplify, a 30-year-old female weighing approximately 150 lbs while running at a pace of a 10-minute mile for 1 hour will burn about 135 calories/hour more than if she were just walking.[9] That is a lot of effort to equal the calories in 1.5 apples, yet many athletes will perform exercise at that intensity, and then consume 1000 calories or more extra from a sports drink thinking that they already "burned it off." This also does not take into account that the same person would have burned about 71 calories during the same time period if he or she were just sleeping.

The Facts

In order to maximize calorie burning and metabolism, increasing lean muscle tissue is the most beneficial way to "burn extra calories." There may be a threshold where elite athletes are able to in effectively eat whatever they want, but their training regimens are well beyond what the majority of competitive athletes (nevermind lay-people) would endure.

The Myth: You Can Only Use 30 Grams of Protein From a Meal

This myth is easily debunked based on a contradiction in government recommendations. The USDA guidelines for protein intake are 1.4 to 2.2g/kg of body weight. For a bodybuilder weighing 275 lbs, that translates to up to 275 g of protein necessary per day. While the absolute recommendation may be appropriate (depending on the source, and it is a controversial subject), it becomes difficult to explain how to incorporate that if the body can only process 30 g at a time. That implies that the bodybuilder would have to eat at least 9 separate meals of 30 g of protein each day to maintain his muscle mass, and does not explain how much time is necessary in between meals to constitute a separate feeding. Certainly, that is not a daily regimen that would be easy to keep up with, and many athletes only eat 2 to 5 meals per day maximum.

The Facts

Protein intake recommendations vary based on lean tissue, type and intensity of activity involved on a daily basis, and goals of the individual. Guidelines should only be used as such, and normal protein intake should be calculated based on the amount of lean tissue an individual has, not his or her total weight.

The Myth: High-Protein Diet Strains Kidney Function

Since one of the main biological roles of the kidneys is to excrete and metabolize nitrogen byproducts from the protein that is eaten, it was believable that eating more protein will "strain" the kidneys in otherwise healthy people due to the excess workload that extra protein would cause by ingestion. This is similar to the argument made against acid-forming diets; however, there is no such research to support this, and there is quite a bit of evidence debunking it. The brain has specific mechanisms that regulate the desire for protein, and these mechanisms are difficult to override through shear willpower.[10]

Furthermore, no study that has postulated that "excess" protein intake will strain the kidneys has any objective qualification for that definition. We do not know if the term *excess protein* means 10% more than the government recommendations, 20% more, etc. We also have never clearly defined what a "strain" on the kidneys means. It could be a positive nitrogen balance, however, that is a common occurrence even when people eat a large steak, and the detrimental effects of that have not been substantiated.

The Facts

If we want to vindicate or convict protein, we must study its effects on healthy kidneys. We have to see if it specifically creates problems rather than potentially worsens them. According to the analysis of Martin et al, there exists no evidence that protein intake negatively impacts renal health in otherwise healthy, active individuals. There is some evidence that already impaired renal function might worsen with increased protein, but you cannot apply that logic with everyone, regardless of renal health.[11,12]

Simply put, healthy kidneys can handle plenty of protein. It is one of their primary functions.

The Myth: Saturated Fat Increases Blood Cholesterol and Risk of Heart Disease

Humans have been eating saturated fat in large quantities since humans have been eating. It was demonized years ago by the landmark "Seven Countries Study,"[13] an observational study that claimed that saturated fat was the cause of heart disease and cancer. It has since been criticized for its outlandish claims, stretched extrapolations, incorrect conclusions, and omitted data, including the fact that there are countries where people eat a lot of fat but have little heart disease, such as Holland and Norway, as well as countries that eat very little fat and have a lot of heart disease, such as Chile. The same authors even went as far as to say later on that "there is no evidence that any of the observed cancer-serum cholesterol relationships among or within the populations involve an effect of serum cholesterol concentration on oncogenesis or cancer mortality."[14]

Cholesterol is found in the membrane of every single cell in the body, helping to regulate structure and function. Cholesterol is also used to make steroid hormones like cortisol, testosterone, estrogen, and the active form of Vitamin D.

About 80% of the cholesterol in our bodies is actually produced by our own cells in the liver, and every cell in the body can produce cholesterol. The cholesterol we eat is usually a minor source compared to the amount we produce—about 20% total.[15]

The Fact

Not only do saturated fats raise the good type of cholesterol (**high-density lipo-proteins** [HDL] cholesterol), saturated fats also only mildly elevate **low-density lipoproteins** (LDL).[16,17] This may sound like there is still a large problem elevating LDL; however, there are 2 subtypes of LDL: small and dense or large.[18,19] Small and dense LDL particles can become mischievous by sticking to arterial walls and causing inflammation; however, saturated fats only elevate the large, fluffy LDL particles, which are benign and can even be beneficial.[20,21]

Saturated fats are given an incorrect stigma by poor research and USDA recommendations, but a simple review of that research will show how wrong that stigma is and that we need to be better educated on nutrition mechanisms.

The Myth: Sports Drinks Are a Great Way to Improve Energy During Physical Activity

You can find various sports drinks at just about any convenience store, gym, or university, as well all over media with advertisements explaining how important they are for recovery, energy, and replacing electrolytes. A simple understanding of glucose metabolism will show that sports drinks are largely unnecessary at best, and dangerous at worst.

Sports drinks for the purposes of this text are any drink designed or marketed for consumption during or after strenuous activity or exercise. They typically contain certain electrolytes as well as a high amount of sugar.

In order to properly break down any manufacturer claims on the benefits of sports drinks, it is important to note that any effect of a sports drink is also dependent on the context of the athlete's diet as a whole. The majority of research comparing sports drinks to water or other drinks does not take this into account and is likely the most important aspect when trying to show a marked difference in performance.

Humans utilize glycogen (the storage form of glucose) from 3 sources: muscle, liver, and blood. Transportation of liver glycogen is dependent on levels of **insulin** and **glucagon**. When glucagon is present, the liver dumps glycogen into the blood stream in order to be used as energy. For this to happen, blood sugar and insulin levels must be low.

Insulin has the opposite effect. When we ingest carbs or large amounts of protein, they cause a concomitant release of insulin from the pancreas, which, in turn, causes a cascade of hormonal responses. These responses create an internal environment that make it difficult to utilize glycogen from the liver or muscles. In order for muscles to have access to muscle or liver glycogen, insulin levels must be low.[22]

The importance of the relationship between insulin, glucagon, glycogen, and adrenaline cannot be overstated. In order to access muscle and liver glycogen stores, insulin needs to be low.[23,24] This is precisely why when marathon runners "hit the wall," they believe that they have run out of glycogen stores and therefore have no more energy to run. However, several studies have shown through muscle biopsies taken from marathon runners who say they cannot continue close to the end of a race that the runners actually still have plenty of glycogen stores left. The reason why they "hit the wall" is because they do not have the ability to access those stores due to high insulin levels from ingesting things like sports drinks or gels, and the carbs from those supplements have not had enough time to process in order to keep up with the physical demand of the body.

The Facts

While sports drinks can benefit certain athletes in specific situations depending on the context of their diet, physical activity type, and intensity, the vast majority of athletes would not benefit from drinking sports drinks in general. In many cases, they can actually be detrimental to the athlete at best, and harmful at worst.

The Myth: Eating Six Meals Per Day Improves Metabolism

TEF is the amount of energy expenditure above the resting metabolic rate due to the cost of processing food for use and storage. Every time you ingest food, metabolic rate increases slightly for a few hours. Ironically, it takes energy to break down and absorb energy. The amount of energy expended is directly proportional to the amount of calories and nutrients consumed in the meal.

As an example, if we measure TEF for a 2400-calorie diet over a 24-hour period with 30% protein, 40% carb, and 30% fat macronutrient breakdown, we can run a trial of the following variable meal frequency:

* 3 meals: 800 kcal/meal
* 6 meals: 400 kcal/meal
* 10 meals: 240 kcal/meal

In example 1, we would see a larger and long-lasting boost in metabolic rate that would gradually taper off until the next time food is consumed. Example 2 would yield a more steady boost in metabolic rate, and example 3 would be somewhere in the middle.

The salient point between these different examples is that, at the end of that specific 24-hour period, there would be no difference in total TEF. Meal frequency is not affected by it.

A very high-quality review of meal frequency studies showed that "studies using whole-body calorimetry and doubly labelled water to assess total 24 [hour] energy expenditure find no difference between nibbling and gorging."[25]

The Facts

It is perplexing why some nutrition professionals keep repeating the myth of "stoking the metabolic fire" by eating small meals very frequently. It is most likely that the concept of TEF is not well understood and some may have disregarded the essential point that TEF is proportional to the calories consumed in each meal.

It is also possible that the origin of this myth is based on some epidemiological studies that found an inverse correlation between high meal frequency and body weight in the study subjects. Unfortunately, those studies did not control for calorie intake and were not performed on a physically active population. This does not mean that certain individuals would not benefit from smaller, more frequent meals during the day. Some athletes may find it prevents from overeating, keeps their calories on track, prevents hunger pangs, or is just a preference based on their schedule.

HOW TO LOOK AT NEW INFORMATION

There is a saying that goes "correlation does not imply causation," and this requires further explanation since it explains many myths about nutrition. Just because there is a correlation between eating fewer meals during the day and higher rates of obesity, that does not mean that eating few meals causes obesity. Epidemiological studies like this do not take into account that people who eat infrequently and are obese also are of the personality type that skips breakfast and has 2 donuts and a large coffee with extra sugar on their way to work in the morning, is too busy to eat much during the day, and then overeats at night. They also tend to be unconcerned about their diet.

It is also important to remember that people who begin eating a low meal frequency diet are also actively trying to lose weight, and therefore will be starting at a higher weight initially. The overriding point is that the correlation between meal frequency and obesity is that of a behavioral pattern and not a causal relationship.

Epidemiology is of course necessary during the scientific process to determine causal patterns; however, epidemiology only provides investigators with a question, not an answer. If we see that people who eat less frequently tend to be more obese, we should then ask why that happens and not jump to any conclusions. Unfortunately, much of the current USDA guidelines are based on poor epidemiological evidence, such as the China study and Seven Countries study.

The China study results recommend veganism (no animal-based food whatsoever), and that is the healthiest way to eat for humans. These results are not even supported by the author's own data. For example, the author of the China study collected data from, but does not mention in his results, the county of Tuoli in China. The inhabitants in Tuoli ate 45% of their diet as fat, 134 g of animal protein each day (twice as much as the average American), and rarely ate vegetables or other plant foods. Yet, according to the data direct from the study, they were extremely healthy with low rates of heart disease and cancer; healthier, in fact, than many of the counties that were vegan or nearly vegan. This is just one of many cases of the selective citation and data cherry-picking the author employs in the China study.[26]

The Seven Countries study may be more important as it has very well shaped the world's fear of fat and potentially set nutrition science backward more than 50 years. A full criticism of the study is beyond the scope of this text, but the largest criticism shows why epidemiological data can only bring questions to the forefront, and answer them. The reason why it is named the "Seven" Countries study is because the author, Ancel Keyes, studied 7 countries in Europe and showed a correlation between heart disease, blood lipids, and increased fat intake, shown in Figure 3-1.[27]

While this graph may look compelling, Keyes did not mention that he did not study 7 countries. He studied 22 countries and eliminated the data from the countries that did not fit his hypothesis. You can see from the graph in Figure 3-2 what it would look like if you include all 22 countries, and the results are all over the place.

It is important to note that the correlation of increased fat intake and heart disease risk did not fully go away, but again, correlation does not mean causation.

Something very important to consider when researching nutrition is that the vast majority of nutrition research is not about what people eat, it is about what people tell us they eat. Historically, people are very bad at estimating calorie intake.[28] Even dietitians, when compared to non-dietitians in terms of food intake, can be off by 10% or more.[29] Unless a well-controlled study is performed in a controlled environment like a metabolic ward, it is very difficult to trust study findings without being able to replicate them later under the same conditions, and that can be costly. That is why it is imperative to be able to not only fully digest all of the data from a research study, and it is even more important to be able to think critically about what the results imply.

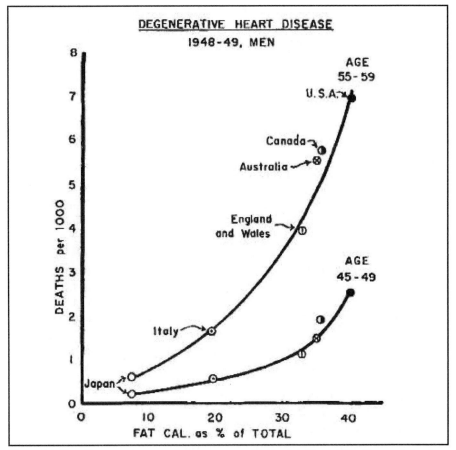

Figure 3-1. Mortality rate as compared to percentage of fat in diet. (Reprinted with permission from Atherosclerosis: a problem in newer public health. *J Mt Sinai Hosp N Y.* 1953;20(2):118-139.)

Figure 3-2. Mortality from arterio-sclerotic and degenerative heart disease and percent of total calories from fat, males ages 55 to 59 years. (Reprinted from Yerushalmy J, Hilleboe HE. Fat in the diet and mortality from heart disease; a methodologic note. *N Y State J Med.* 1957;57:2343-2354.)

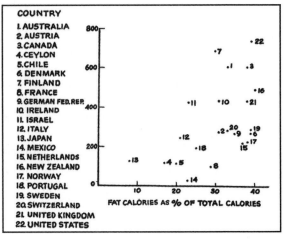

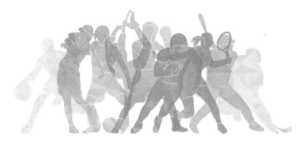

DEFINITIONS

Ketogenic diet: A low-carb diet where the body produces ketones in the liver to be used as energy; a typical breakdown of a ketogenic diet is 80% fat, 15% protein, and 5% carbohydrate

High-density lipoproteins: Lipoprotein is often referred to as "good" cholesterol; HDL picks up excess cholesterol in your blood and takes it back to your liver where it is broken down and removed from your body

Low-density lipoproteins: Lipoprotein that transports cholesterol from the liver to the tissues of the body; it is therefore considered the "bad" cholesterol

Insulin: A hormone produced in the pancreas by the islets of Langerhans that regulate the amount of glucose in the blood

Glucagon: A peptide hormone produced by alpha cells of the pancreas; it works to raise the concentration of glucose and fat in the bloodstream

REFERENCES

1. Feinman RD, Fine EJ. "A calorie is a calorie" violates the second law of thermodynamics. *Nutrition Journal.* 2004;3:9.
2. Atwater WO, Woods CD. The availability and fuel values of food materials. In *Connecticut (Storrs) Agricultural Experiment Station 12th Annual Report.* Storrs, CT: Storrs Agricultural Experiment Station; 1900:73-123.
3. Jequier E. Pathways to obesity. *Int J Obes Relat Metab Disord.* 2002;26(Suppl2):S12-S17.
4. Lindeberg S, Ahrén B, Nilsson A, et al. Determinants of serum triglycerides and high-density lipoprotein cholesterol in traditional Trobriand Islanders: the Kitava study. *Scand J Clin Lab Invest.* 2003;63(3):175-180.
5. Hatzis CM, Sifaki-Pistolla D, Papandreou C, et al. Validity of the cohort of Crete in the Seven Countries Study: a time-series study applied to the cancer mortality trend between 1960 and 2011. *Oncol Lett.* 2013;5(3):964-968.
6. Kiefer J. Introduction. *Carb Backloading.* 2012:19.
7. Doris S, Chan M, Lau R, et al. Red and processed meat and colorectal cancer incidence: meta-analysis of prospective studies. *PLoS One.* 2011;6(6):e20456.
8. Barr SB, Wright JC. Postprandial energy expenditure in whole-food and processed-food meals: implications for daily energy expenditure. *Food Nutr Res.* 2010;54:10.

9.   Wilkin LD, Cheryl A, Haddock BL. Energy expenditure comparison between walking and running in average fitness individuals. *J Strength Cond Res.* 2012;26(4): 1039-1044.

10. Morrison CD, Reed SD, Henagan TM. Homeostatic regulation of protein intake: in search of a mechanism. *Am J Physiol Regul Integr Comp Physiol.* 2012;302(8):R917-R928.

11. Manninen A. High-protein weight loss diets and purported adverse effects: where is the evidence? *J Int Soc Sports Nutr.* 2004;1(1):45-51.

12. Martin W, Armstrong L, Rodriguez N. Dietary protein intake and renal function. *Nutr Metab (Lond).* 2005;2:25.

13. Menotti A, Keys A, Aravanis C, et al. Seven countries study: first 20-year mortality data in 12 cohorts of six countries. *Ann Med.* 1989;21(3):175-179.

14. Keys A, Aravanis C, Blackburn H, et al. Serum cholesterol and cancer mortality in the Seven Countries Study. *Am J Epidemiol.* 1985;121(6):870-883.

15. Daniels T, Killinger K, Michal J, et al. Lipoproteins, cholesterol homeostasis and cardiac health. *Int J Biol Sci.* 2009;5(5):474-488.

16. Morris JN, Marr J, Heady J. Diet and plasma cholesterol in 99 bank men. *Br Med J.* 1963;1(5330):571-576.

17. Nichols AB, Ravenscroft C, Lamphiear DE, et al. Daily nutritional intake and serum lipid levels. The Tecumseh study. *Am J Clin Nutr.* 1976;29(12):1384-1392.

18. Packard C, Caslake M, Shepherd J, et al. The role of small, dense low density lipoprotein (LDL): a new look. *Intl J of Card.* 2000;74(Supplement 1):S17-S22.

19. Gardner C, Fortmann, SP, Krauss RM. Association of small low-density lipoprotein particles with the incidence of coronary artery disease in men and women. *J Am Med Assoc.* 1996;276(11):875-881.

20. Dreon DM, Fernstrom HA, Campos H, et al. Change in dietary saturated fat intake is correlated with change in mass of large low-density-lipoprotein particles in men. *Am J Clin Nutr.* 1998;67(5):828-836.

21. Siri-Tarino PW, Sun Q, Hu FB, et al. Saturated fat, carbohydrate, and cardiovascular disease. *Am J Clin Nutr.* 2010;91(3):502-509.

22. Jensen J, Rustad PI, Kolnes AJ, et al. The role of skeletal muscle glycogen breakdown for regulation of insulin sensitivity by exercise. *Front Physiol.* 2011;2:112.

23. Sherwin RS, Saccà L. Effect of epinephrine on glucose metabolism in humans: contribution of the liver. *Am J Physiol.* 1984;247(2 Pt 1):E157-E165.

24. Malherbe HW, Bone AD. The effect of insulin on the levels of adrenaline and noradrenaline in human blood. *J Endocrinol.* 1954;11:285-297.

25. Cameron JD, Cyr MJ, Doucet E. Increased meal frequency does not promote greater weight loss in subjects who were prescribed an 8-week equi-energetic energy-restricted diet. *Br J Nutr.* 2010;103(8):1098-1101.

26. Campbell TC, Campbell TM. *The China Study: The Most Comprehensive Study of Nutrition Ever Conducted and the Startling Implications for Diet, Weight Loss and Long-Term Health.* Dallas, TX: BenBella Books; 2006.

27. Keys A. *Seven Countries: A Multivariate Analysis of Death and Coronary Heart Disease.* Cambridge, MA: Harvard University Press; 1980.

28. Yanetz R, Kipnis V, Carroll RJ, et al. Using biomarker data to adjust estimates of the distribution of usual intakes for misreporting: application to energy intake in the US population. *J Am Diet Assoc.* 2008;108(3):455-464; discussion 464.

29. Champagne CM, Bray GA, Kurtz AA, et al. Energy intake and energy expenditure: a controlled study comparing dietitians and non-dietitians. *J Am Diet Assoc.* 2002;102(10):1428-1432.

Practitioners need to understand the origins, signs, symptoms, and medical complications of disordered eating and eating disorders in their athletes. By appreciating the medical risks of caloric restriction, purging, and binge eating, practitioners can perform the vital role of early identification and referral to a multidisciplinary team with expertise in eating disorders. Caloric restriction bears the risks of bradycardia or slow heart rate; slowed digestion including gastroparesis and constipation; sex hormone deficiency; bone density loss; and, in more extreme cases, end-organ failure such as hypoglycemia, bone marrow suppression, and liver dysfunction. Purging can result in significant volume depletion, electrolyte abnormalities, and the risk of edema or fluid weight gain upon purging cessation. Binge eating disorder can be missed due to size stigma in the medical field and lack of awareness of this being a full-fledged eating disorder.

Disordered Eating and Eating Disorders in Athletes

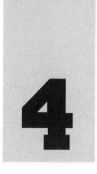

Jennifer L. Gaudiani, MD, CEDS, FAED

Key Takeaways

* Understand the signs, symptoms, and treatment protocols for various eating disorders in order to properly designate care.
* Body composition is not the "end-all" for overall health.
* Malnutrition can happen to athletes of any shape or size.
* Mental illness is a large part of the origin of disordered eating and must be treated on an individual basis.
* Practitioners should never feel pressured to treat disordered eating by themselves. A team approach of multiple disciplines is best.

Food is the vital fuel that permits athletes to train and perform. Regardless of their sport, athletes are bombarded with a bewildering variety of social messages about "healthy eating." Some principles are sound, while others veer toward pseudoscience or are frankly dangerous. Those in the latter category tend to promote a causative association between categories of nutrition and disease states or performance boosts that have little or no bearing on reality or science. In this chapter, starting from the premise that athletes are susceptible to nutrition and performance messages, I will review how this makes them vulnerable to significantly disordered eating patterns. Disordered eating invariably leads to worse athletic performance, even if it might help in the short term, and can furthermore cause a number of medical problems not well recognized even by medical doctors. Even worse, disordered eating can lead to full-blown eating disorders, which carry the highest death rate of any mental illness.

Amato D. *An Athletic Trainer's Guide to Sports Nutrition (pp 45-63).*
© 2019 SLACK Incorporated.

By understanding the clinical presentations of disordered eating and eating disorders, and the medical complications that arise from them, the practitioner can play a vital role in early identification and referral to an expert multidisciplinary outpatient team. In addition, they can hold themselves and their profession to a high standard of scientific, evidence-based teachings about nutrition and performance.

Let us start with the "unwinnable game" of body composition and shape these days. In a sport where being big and strong matters? You'll never get big enough. Where leanness and muscularity is prized? Someone else always seems to be more cut. Where being strong but light is a must? Each year, somehow someone taller and bigger is scrambling to make weight. Our commercial society thrives on exposing insecurities and then selling people the solution. Women have of course been fielding this technique for generations, with ads reminding them that their hair/skin/body is inadequate (but if they buy this product, they will improve and so will their lives). We see evidence of this strategy creeping into the domain of boys and men too, now. Action figures from the 1970s that had normal body proportions are remade currently as steroidal, grotesque versions of the same character, with bulging muscles, zero body fat, and tiny waists. Indeed, even our boys' Halloween costumes unfortunately perpetuate these messages, as preschoolers wear superhero costumes padded with deltoids, biceps, pectoral muscles, and a 6 pack. This contributes from early on to a subtle, but real, message that our little boys cannot be super or magical unless they have the "right" body for it.

Athletes are particularly susceptible to food messages. They are hard-working, not afraid of pain, and willing to suffer for improved results. They trust coaching relationships that may work great on the field, road, or stage, but may not serve them well with nutritional advice. Practitioners can help empower athletes to request that nutrition recommendations come from experts—typically sports or eating disorder nutritionists—rather than coaches, who are surely well-meaning but may not have scientifically sound perspectives. It is very important that athletes hear that requesting this expertise is not being "uncoachable," but rather responsible.

Athletes want what is best for their bodies and are always looking for the "edge" over the competition. Modern society often suggests that can be found through a change in food intake. Of course, the best "edge" is almost certainly obtained through careful attention to good hydration, consistent sleep and adequate recovery time, sufficient energy intake, and attention to one's mental health and emotional needs. Without these to recharge and heal the body and mind, training and performance strategy will be much less effective, and engagement in fad food philosophies will not help at all. It is always worth thinking about diverse populations and risk. The pressure to attain perfection may be even higher in racially diverse and LBGTQ+ athletes.

The problem lies in the fact that size, shape, leanness, and muscularity are still overvalued in sports, even when it comes to refereed as opposed to judged sports. As a result, to honor the high-performance vehicle that is the self, and to try and optimize performance, athletes can apply stringent criteria to their food intake that can actually lead to malnourishment, medical problems, and mental illness, endpoints that are anything but healthy and optimal. Many modern "healthy eating" recommendations are unscientific fads that are unhelpful at best or harmful and even actively dangerous to the health at worst. They might be labeled, "all pain, no gain." A great example of this is so-called "clean eating." Beautiful, locally sourced, organic, and colorful fresh foods are terrific to eat, of course. However, human bodies are exquisitely designed to make effective use of a remarkably broad array of nutrients, and thrive. Unlike cows or whales that have to eat a huge amount of a very few types of food, humans can grow from babies into adults on a wide variety of foods. We know this looking around the globe and seeing how differently people eat in various geographies. Despite this fact, clean eating followers come to believe that anything else somehow will sully the temple of the body, or promote "inflammation" and disease processes. On the contrary, I like to think of the human body as being the ultimate off-roading nutritional machine. Getting obsessed with clean eating is like getting into peak athletic shape and never leaving the house for fear of getting muddy. It imagines a risk that simply does not exist, and that puts unnecessary limits on the amazing body.

The diet mentality is not without risk. Getting into an overly rigid relationship with food can turn into disordered eating or a full-blown eating disorder. Why play that game of Roulette? We know from sports psychology that visualization matters. When athletes become too focused on and fearful of food, they spend a lot of time each day considering the next meal, the last meal, food prep, and social eating, regardless of whether they are trying to change their weight or size. They are essentially visualizing themes that are negative, rigid, and anxious. This will not help their performance.

To help athletes avoid food issues altogether or identify those who have gotten in trouble and need expert referrals, practitioners need to know the science of bodies and food. Specifically, what happens medically in malnutrition? Remember, malnutrition can occur at any body shape and size. A linebacker who starves himself all day and then binge eats junk food and drinks at night ravenously only to wake up in shame the next morning and repeat the pattern can become malnourished. Rowers or wrestlers who have to cut weight several times per year can become acutely malnourished, not to mention dehydrated and with dangerous electrolyte abnormalities, depending on what techniques they are using. A cyclist who becomes overly fixated on healthy eating and staying lean during an injury can also become malnourished. The more we understand how the body reacts to a chronic imbalance between energy intake and performative output, the more we can identify and support athletes in need of help.

RESTRICTION OF CALORIES

Case: Lauren

Lauren is a 20-year-old collegiate distance runner. Last year, her times improved as she started following a low-carbohydrate, no-processed-food diet and lost 10 lbs. She was widely praised. In the last 3 months, she has become quite withdrawn, having previously been a leader on her team and someone whom others could turn to. She rarely eats socially anymore. As the season starts, her performance is worse than last year, and her usual level-headedness in the face of challenges has been replaced by a more brittle, self-judging spirit. She pushes herself harder than ever in practice, and in fact has been logging miles that her coaches actively tell her not to. They ask her to see the team dietitian, who recommends easing off the diet. Lauren says she would not mind putting back on some muscle weight, but she makes no dietary changes because she is concerned that any extra food would actually just turn into fat. She also gets full really quickly after just a few bites of food and decides "that must be all my body needs." Constipation is a new issue. A stress fracture just 1 month into the season heightens her practitioner's concern.

The practitioner notes that Lauren looks visibly underweight. Her hands and feet are cold, with bluish-red fingers and toes. She now has fine, soft hair growing on her face. Her pulse is 39 at rest, although right after she arrives in the practitioner's office, having walked down the hall from the locker room, her pulse was over 90. She notes without concern that she has not had a menstrual period in over 1 year, saying that is so typical for the women on her team that she does not give it a second thought. She says she was shaky yesterday morning. She checked her blood sugar with a roommate's glucometer and found it was 50 mg/dL. The shakes went away after she ate some fruit. She has an ache deep in her right groin where her femoral neck stress fracture was diagnosed. The practitioner refers her urgently to a good doctor, known for having expertise with eating disorders and athletes.

––––––––––––––––

The first consideration in understanding Lauren's case is to think about the overall diagnosis, and what might be the implications of this diagnosis as far as outcomes. There are 3 possibilities: orthorexia nervosa, anorexia nervosa (AN), or atypical AN. The first diagnosis does not exist officially in the **Diagnostic and Statistical Manual of Mental Disorders** (DSM-V), the book that defines mental illnesses.[1] However, it can be thought of as a potential "gateway disorder" to the DSM-V eating disorders, so it is worth practitioners' awareness.

Orthorexia nervosa is a term coined by Steven Bratman.[2] It refers to a person who is intrusively obsessed with eating in a healthy manner. Someone with orthorexia spends so much time thinking about, choosing, and preparing healthy foods that it interferes with other aspects of life. Feelings of impurity, disgust, and guilt follow consumption of food not regarded as healthy. The person's sense of safety, self-esteem, and peace are overly dependent on the purity of what is eaten. To make this unofficial diagnosis, one must have food rules and preoccupations about healthy eating, including use of specific supplements. These food rules and constructions of healthy eating may vary widely from one person with orthorexia to another. Furthermore, the compulsive behavior and preoccupations must become clinically impairing.[3] That is, it is not just that someone becomes hyperfocused on food, but rather that this focus negatively impacts a person's social, athletic, academic, or professional functioning. Orthorexia nervosa can lead to life-threatening malnutrition.[4] Without ever intending to lose weight, and without any distortions in their perception of body shape or size, a patient may follow his or her particular food rules to the point where he or she becomes medically compromised and emaciated. In addition, a chronically restrictive mindset can lead to bingeing or chewing and spitting, as the hungry individual's mind becomes ravenous for off-limits food groups and sufficient calories. Athletes' shame, isolation, and reluctance to discuss these breaches in their food rules and self-care may cause them not to discuss such behaviors and, as a result, they miss out on needed help.

AN is a DSM-V diagnosis. It comes in 2 subtypes: restrictive (AN-R) and binge-purge (AN-BP). For a diagnosis of AN, patients must show a restriction of energy intake leading to a low body weight, fear of gaining weight and of food, and a distortion in the perception of one's body image. The presence or absence of menstrual periods are no longer a criterion for the diagnosis of AN in the DSM-V. AN-R refers to patients who purely restrict calories without ever purging them. Those with AN-R may also engage in excessive or compulsive exercise. AN-BP refers to those who restrict calories and also purge, whether they engage in bingeing or not. They, too, may use exercise in the service of their eating disorder. Those with AN always have a low body weight for height, by definition. By contrast, as per a different case described later, patients with bulimia nervosa are typically of normal or higher body weight.

AN carries the highest mortality of any mental illness; 5% to 20% of patients with AN will die from it, half from medical causes and half from suicide as it is a punishingly cruel disease emotionally. Those with AN have a 6x mortality rate compared with their age-matched peers.[5] An estimated 90% of those with AN are female, and 0.5% to 1% of American women have AN. It carries a grim prognosis. Fewer than 50% recover, while about 30% improve but never get completely better, and 20% develop a severe and enduring form of the illness, which is devastating to patients and their families financially and in terms of inability to achieve academic, professional, and interpersonal milestones.[6] Despite these sobering and, to many people, surprising statistics, full recovery from AN is possible.

AN is not a "choice" picked by a young, white, wealthy girl as a means of attention-getting, as has unfortunately been a pervasive misconception. Rather, it is a complicated physiological, psychological, and sociological problem that affects people of all ages, genders, races, and socioeconomic levels. It has a strong genetic component because temperamental traits are inherited from the parents that appear to predispose patients to developing AN. These include intelligence, anxiety, perfectionism, rigidity, determination, and sensitivity to external validation or invalidation. These traits are productive, positive traits usually, and they can certainly drive athletes to work hard and perform well. However, when the temperamental traits are unusually pronounced and are located within a thin-obsessed society, simple weight loss of any kind—whether from a diet, an intention to eat healthier food, or a medical illness that causes weight loss—can trigger the onset of a full-blown eating disorder.

The third diagnosis we will consider in Lauren is atypical AN. This, too, is a formal diagnosis in the DSM-V. It applies to patients who show all of the symptoms and fears of classical AN, but without concurrent low body weight. Because doctors unfortunately bring significant weight bias and stigma to the bedside, patients with atypical anorexia may be missed or even praised for weight loss, especially when they

TABLE 4-1

COMPARISON OF DIAGNOSTIC CRITERIA FOR ORTHOREXIA NERVOSA, ANOREXIA NERVOSA, AND ATYPICAL ANOREXIA NERVOSA PER DSM-V

CRITERION	ORTHOREXIA NERVOSA	ANOREXIA NERVOSA	ATYPICAL ANOREXIA NERVOSA
Formal DSM-V diagnosis	No	Yes	Yes
Restriction of energy intake (calories)	Sometimes	Yes	Yes
Excessive exercise	Can occur	Can occur	Can occur
Intense fear of gaining weight or becoming fat	No	Yes	Yes
Distortion in perception of body weight, body shape, or severity of disease	No	Yes	Yes
Significantly low body weight	No	Yes	No
Hyperfocus on quality or purity of food	Yes	Can occur	Can occur
Purging (vomiting, laxatives, or diuretics)	No	In binge-purge subtype	Can occur

start with a larger body size.[7,8] However, because significant, rapid weight loss can cause medical complications just as serious as prolonged low body weight, diagnosis and expert referral are just as vital for these patients. In Lauren's case, what started as a desire for improved performance through dietary finessing progressed to orthorexia nervosa and then to AN-R (Table 4-1).

The prevalence of disordered eating in athletes is dependent upon the sport. Among adult and adolescent female elite athletes, the prevalence of disordered eating is about 20% and 13%, respectively, while among adult and adolescent male athletes, prevalence is 8% and 3%, respectively.[9,10] Broadly speaking, sports that are judged bring higher risks of disordered eating than sports that are refereed, and sports with a thin/lean aesthetic carry higher risks yet. Practitioners may wonder how to distinguish an athlete with disordered eating from one who accidentally went too far down the proverbial rabbit hole of food rules in the quest for improved performance. When a practitioner encounters an athlete with medical, emotional, or sports-affecting nutritional issues, they can ask themselves, "Is this individual driven to win, or driven by fear?" The athlete who is driven to win and who does not have an eating disorder will follow a nutritionist's recommendations, increase calories and body weight, and rest as advised. They recognize that in their passionate quest for an edge, they accidentally went too far and they willingly and promptly change their behaviors. The athlete who is driven by fear, usually the fear engendered by the distortions of a growing mental illness, will say they will follow recommendations but find they cannot. Their drive for thinness, fear of weight gain, body image disturbance, and fear of further loss of performance will maintain the eating disordered behaviors. Regardless of their eloquent, articulate arguments why they are not "sick enough" to foster such concerns in their teammates and practitioners, the fact is that they continue to restrict calories and overexert their bodies. Denial is a hallmark of eating disorders, and one cannot wait to intervene until a patient shows up realizing he or she has a problem and asking for help.

Let us turn to a review of all the medical problems Lauren has developed as a result of her AN. Broadly speaking, the human brain responds to starvation by slowing the metabolism. The physiologic changes experienced by someone with a chronic imbalance of energy intake and energy output are now characterized by the syndrome Relative Energy Deficiency in Sport (or RED-S). RED-S replaces the Female Athlete Triad, which was limited to females and only focused on the axis of bone density, menstrual regularity, and energy availability. RED-S provides a vastly more encompassing and thorough perspective, highlighting all of the issues related to body and food and sport. It includes impaired physiologic functioning related to metabolic rate, menstrual function, bone health, immunity, protein synthesis, cardiovascular health, gastrointestinal function, psychological impact, and more, in the context of chronic relative energy deficiency.[11]

Mammals must keep their body temperatures even and warm. However, in the face of chronic caloric deprivation, the body tries to spare the number of calories spent on this task. It does so by regrowing fetal hair, called *lanugo*, on the face, a literal pelt that aims to prevent heat loss from the head. It shuts down the microcirculation of the hands and feet so that calorie-warmed blood does not get cool circulating through the extremities. This is called *acrocyanosis*, or "blue tips" of the fingers and toes. Patients feel chilly all the time and seek warmer clothing.

Lauren's pulse has dropped to the mid-30s at rest, and she interprets this as being a manifestation of her athletic heart. However, you noted that with minimal ambulation, her pulse was up in the 90s as she entered the office. A true athlete's heart remains slow (although perhaps not in the 30s) with minimal exertion because it is a well-fed, robust machine. A starving person, however, slows the heart rate at rest like that of a hibernating bear, with high vagal or parasympathetic tone, so as not to waste a calorie on an extra beat of the heart at rest. However, with minimal exertion, the heart rate might go up by 75% or more because the body recognizes it has lost muscle mass through starvation and is, physiologically, deconditioned. I recommend this "walk across the room test" to all practitioners as they assess whether an athlete has bradycardia from fitness or from malnutrition.

Lauren's hypoglycemia is her most medically concerning finding. Hypoglycemia is probably the killer in AN-R, not cardiac complications. With rare exceptions, the brain can only run on glucose. Glucoses less than 70 mg/dL are low. Since the body is exceptionally efficient in storing glucose, we have only about 5 g of glucose circulating in our blood, or about 20 kcals. We store about 2000 kcals in glycogen in our liver and muscles. In someone who is chronically undereating relative to caloric burn, the body uses up these stores quite quickly. Thereafter, in the absence of consumed carbs, the body is forced to break down its own lean muscle mass to synthesize glucose, using fat as the energy source to do this. This is a powerful reminder that practitioners can bring to their athletes: significant exercise while malnourished does not "tone" or "elongate" muscles, it shrinks them. Because our lean muscle mass is a major driver of our metabolism, all that athletes are doing is slowing their own metabolisms by restricting and exercising. When the body can no longer break down enough muscle to satisfy the brain's needs, blood glucose levels fall and hypoglycemia develops. Severe or persistent enough hypoglycemia will cause cardiac arrest. It is a serious sign of malnutrition.

Lauren's early fullness and constipation are further signs of a slowed metabolism. Her brain has slowed her digestion to spare calories. *Gastroparesis* refers to the loss of normal stomach peristalsis, or smooth muscle movements, that passes ingested food forward into the small intestine. Nearly universal in caloric restriction and rapid weight loss, regardless of body size, this needs to be assessed and treated by a doctor and dietitian in tandem. It causes early fullness, nausea, and bloating. Gastroparesis will almost always resolve with nutritional rehabilitation, but often prescription medicines are needed to permit that rehabilitation process to proceed smoothly. Constipation occurs by the same mechanism and is a sign of malnourishment.

Menstrual period loss in females reflects an overall process in which sex hormones revert to the pre-pubertal state in the setting of malnourishment. Similarly, in males, testosterone drops. Broadly speaking, our brain understands that this is not a body that is safe to produce children. In females, the ovaries and uterus can shrink, returning to their pre-adolescent size. Sex drive falls as well. The more researchers study the issue of sex hormones in malnutrition, the more we understand that, as with many combinations of genetic predisposition and environmental trigger, patients vary widely. In one study, 38% of patients presenting for eating disorder treatment were found to have lost their menstrual period while still at a normal body mass index (BMI),[12] while in another, 25% of patients still had their period or regained it while still at a critically low BMI of 14 kg/m^2.[13]

Primary amenorrhea refers to patients never having had a first menstrual period. Secondary amenorrhea refers to patients who at one point had periods, but who now do not. In athletes, primary amenorrhea was diagnosed in 7% of collegiate athletes overall, and in up to 22% of those engaging in sports such as cheerleading, diving, and gymnastics. Presumably, the low body fat and focus on the thin ideal in those sports never fully permitted young women to mature hormonally. Secondary amenorrhea was found in 2% to 5% of collegiate athletes, but in long-distance runners and dancers, the prevalence was 65% to 70%.[11] Hypothalamic hypogonadism causing secondary amenorrhea is the proper way to refer to a regression of the sex hormone axis in response to malnutrition.

So, what is the problem with a chronically low estrogen level in females, or a chronically low testosterone level in males? The main problem is that these states contribute to rapid, severe, and potentially permanent bone density loss when paired with the physiological stressors of chronic malnutrition, typically specifically in the context of low body weight. Most of our bone mass is accrued during adolescence. For those who develop an eating disorder during those years, the mineralization of the skeleton never occurs. In those who develop an eating disorder later, bone density loss can be remarkably rapid, with so-called 75-year-old bones in a 22-year-old athlete.

A **DEXA bone density scan** should be performed within 6 months of menstrual period loss in females and as soon as low body weight or symptoms of low testosterone are a concern in males. The medical nomenclature does not help communicate the urgency and severity to patients who are looking for examples of how they are "fine" and do not need to change their behaviors. In adults over 50 years old, the T-score is used in the DEXA results. A T-score higher than -1 is normal, a score from -1 to -2.5 defines osteopenia, and a score less than -2.5 defines osteoporosis. However, in patients under 50 years old, a different scoring system applies. The Z-score is used instead of the T-score. The results are recorded as "normal" until the Z-score is less than -2, at which point it is only called "below the expected range for age." If a patient between the ages of 20 and 50 has a Z-score of less than -2.0 and has a fragility fracture or secondary cause of bone density loss (like AN), he or she is diagnosed with osteoporosis. In children and adolescents, only if the Z-score is less than -2 and the individual has had a vertebral fracture, 2 long bone fractures by age 10 years, or 3+ long bone fractures by age 19 years, is the diagnosis osteoporosis used.[14]

The problem with this is that, practically, a Z-score of -1.8 in a 20-year-old patient absolutely is not clinically normal, especially if that individual is an athlete who should have extra strong bone density as a result of high-intensity, weightbearing exercise. This highlights the importance of working with physicians who are familiar with eating disorder and athlete physiology and can look beyond the standard radiographic algorithm to interpret a DEXA in a way that is relevant and motivating to the patient. DEXAs should be checked every 2 years after the initial one. An important study found that girls and young women with AN have a 60% increase in fractures compared with age-matched controls, even before bone scans showed reduced bone mineral density. The higher risk was observed as early as 1 year into the diagnosis of AN, and the results were independent of exercise performed.[15]

The gold standard for arresting bone density loss, and perhaps for regaining some bone density, is nutritional rehabilitation and full weight restoration. While the topic of identifying a target weight range is beyond the scope of this chapter, it should generally take into account pre-eating disorder weight, familial body type, menstrual history, pediatric growth percentiles, and a thoughtful ongoing assessment of the whole person. One thing is clear: every day that someone is underweight and has low sex hormone levels, they lose more bone density.[16] Calcium at 1000 to 1500 mg/day and 800 IU/day of vitamin D, keeping levels of Vitamin D-OH at 20 to 30, is appropriate but is not sufficient to treat bone density loss.[17]

A detailed description of the pharmacologic treatment of bone density loss in malnutrition, either in the context of RED-S or AN, is beyond the scope of this chapter, but it is worth mentioning oral contraceptive pills. They have been proven, without a doubt, not to work for bone density loss. Generating a chemical period every month can also cause a woman to minimize the significance of her hypothalamic hypogonadism. Despite this, oral contraceptive pills continue to be mis-prescribed for this indication.

However, transdermal estrogen patches, which are absorbed differently (and do not prevent pregnancy), have now become a vital tool in bone density loss in females with underweight and amenorrhea. Their efficacy has been proven in adolescent girls who have a bone age of at least 15 years and who have a bone mineral density score of less than -2.0, and it may take some time to gain and sustain a normal body weight. A 17-b estradiol patch of 100 mcg twice weekly, with cyclic oral medroxyprogesterone 10 mg/day on days 20 to 30 every month for uterine lining protection, increased bone accrual rates at the spine and hip in adolescents with AN. These are used as a bridge to full weight restoration.[18] New data are emerging that estrogen patches are appropriate for female athletes with amenorrhea and bone density loss, producing both improvements in bone density[19] and even in cognition and memory.[20] An important study found that amenorrheic women with AN who engaged even in moderate exercise—including pacing—had more rapid bone density loss than those who engaged in no exercise. However, once full weight restored, even intensive exercise helped bone density.[21] Appreciating this fact, I nonetheless am convinced that, while serious exercise is a privilege of full recovery, mindful, supervised movement during weight restoration makes recovery sustainable.

Similarly, good screening for bone density loss in male athletes is vital.[22] High-risk populations include those who have low body weights and believe that thinness is correlated with improved running performance[23] and in those with stress fracture history, more than 30 miles of running weekly, and consuming fewer than one calcium-rich food daily.[24] Nutritional rehabilitation and weight restoration is, as with females, the first-line therapy. In males who have completed their linear growth, usually verified by bone age x-ray, have low total testosterone levels, and have low bone density, testosterone replacement via transdermal preparations may be appropriate. The timing of such replacement depends in part on the severity of the bone density loss and possible associated fractures, as well as the length of time expected for weight restoration. Superb criteria exist for determining whether athletes may continue to engage in and compete in their sport, with regard to energy availability and bone density parameters. These are evidence-based and should be promoted wherever possible over less scientific and less rigorous gestalt judgments.[25]

It is worth noting that, although blood tests were not mentioned in Lauren's case, most patients who purely restrict calories will have normal laboratory values. This can confound providers and contribute to denial of illness. However, end-organ damage can occur in rapid weight loss and persistent underweight.[26] Bone marrow failure, called *gelatinous marrow transformation*, can cause low white blood cell counts (leukopenia), low red blood cell counts (anemia), and low platelet counts (thrombocytopenia).[27] Liver damage, with elevations only in the aspartate transaminase and alanine transaminase blood tests, can occur due to cellular apoptosis in response to malnutrition.[28] Skin and hair suffer from poor nutrition, leading to hair loss and fragile skin that tears or bruises easily. Almost without exception, these will all resolve with nutritional rehabilitation.

Resolution of Lauren's Case

At the doctor's office, an electrocardiogram (EKG) and full lab panel are performed, including a complete blood count, complete metabolic panel, vitamin D-OH level, thyroid function tests, prealbumin, and estradiol level. A DEXA bone scan is ordered. The doctor identifies that Lauren has AN and educates her about what that means for her medically. A multidisciplinary team is established that includes Lauren, her doctor, her coach, her athletic trainer, and a dietitian and therapist that have eating disorder expertise. The team offers her the unified message that Lauren must urgently change course and engage in recovery work. She is started on at least 1600 kcals/day with swift escalation, under medical supervision. The team prepares her for the likelihood she will become hypermetabolic during the recovery period and need to consume a remarkably high number of calories/day just to restore the 1 to 2 lbs/week of body weight required. Strict criteria are set for return to running. Lauren is informed that if she is unable to meet the team's weight restoration requirements consistently, she will be referred to a higher level of care.

PURGING

Case: Esteban

Esteban is a 19-year-old freshman wrestler. The transition to college has been a challenging one for him. He is the oldest of his siblings and was always the role model, with high expectations established by his parents. A highly responsible young man, he rarely shares his feelings and instead pushes them down and does whatever has to be done. Moving out of state, settling in to the new academic challenges of college, and establishing himself on his new team have all been more difficult than he would like to admit. However, it does not occur to him to confide in anyone. He thinks he just needs to work through it as he always has.

One night, exhausted from a double practice and faced with school work he had not started, he comes back from team dinner and orders 2 pizzas and devours both, then follows it up with a quart of ice cream, mindlessly eating. Afterward, he feels shocked at himself. Embarrassed and unnerved, he makes himself throw it all up and resolves never to binge or purge again. However, with increasing frequency, he finds himself unable to resist. After bingeing and purging, he does feel a sense of calm, even as he cannot believe what he is doing. The routine of engaging in these behaviors feels like something he can exert control over. He has always had to think about making weight as a wrestler, but he finds himself thinking about weight and food a lot more often.

This season, Esteban had planned to stay at the same weight class as last year, even though he grew 2 inches before college and has become stronger. His teammate's father told him to eat a very low-fat diet to achieve this goal. Between his public low-fat diet and extra running, and his private bingeing and purging, which has extended to include laxative abuse a few days/week, Esteban's weight drops sharply over the next 1.5 months. He does not feel well at all. His trainer had found his body fat at the start of the season to be 13.2%, and now, after a 15-lb weight loss, his body fat is 14.6%.

Around this time, his muscles cramp up severely during practice, and he is escorted to the trainer. Esteban's heart rate is 120 even after resting for a while, his lips and mouth are dry, his blood pressure is low, and his muscles are painfully cramped. On the back of his right hand are a number of small, scabbed scrape marks with calluses, which the trainer recognizes as Russell's sign, from inducing vomiting by manually inducing a gag reflex. Upon compassionate questioning, Esteban admits to his trainer what has been going on. The trainer gets him to urgent care swiftly, concerned about volume depletion and low potassium levels. Indeed, upon testing at urgent care, his potassium level is only 2.9 mEq/L (normal is 3.5 to 5.0), and his bicarbonate is high at 33 mEq/L (normal is 22 to 28), showing severe volume depletion. His QTc interval on his EKG is 495.

Bulimia nervosa is defined by the DSM-V as recurrent episodes of binge eating accompanied by compensatory purging behaviors (vomiting, laxative abuse, or diuretics), occurring at least once per week for 3 months. Patients' sense of self is overly influenced by body shape and weight. Unlike in AN, patients with bulimia nervosa are typically normal weight or higher body weight since usually not all binged calories are fully eliminated (Table 4-2).

The most important medical complications of bulimia nervosa for practitioners to know about are ones related to electrolyte abnormalities and to the cessation of purging. Hypokalemia, or low potassium levels, occur due to loss in vomit, diarrhea, or urine, depending on the type of purging used. Potassium levels less than 3 mEq/L can cause serious medical problems, including muscle cramps or breakdown (rhabdomyolysis), seizure, or cardiac arrest. Hypokalemia can induce a prolonged QTc interval on the EKG, which can progress to torsades de pointes, a terminal cardiac rhythm. QTc intervals are critical and require urgent medical attention when they are greater than 480 in females and greater than 490 in males.

Severe volume depletion, or loss of both salt and water, can occur from all types of purging, but it is most pronounced in those who abuse laxatives due to water losses in diarrhea. Patients who are actively engaged in purging behaviors should be referred to a doctor for regular blood tests, and those with bulimia nervosa, like Esteban, need the same multidisciplinary team that Lauren was referred to. Just because the body weight is not low does not mean there is no danger. As with AN, bulimia nervosa is not a choice that can be fixed through intellectual discussion of the risks. It is a serious mental illness and requires an expert team.

When patients who routinely purge stop purging, whether they have AN or bulimia nervosa, they can rapidly develop edema, or water retention. This can range from

TABLE 4-2	
BULIMIA NERVOSA DIAGNOSTIC CRITERIA PER DSM-V	
CRITERION	**DETAILS**
Recurrent episodes of binge eating	• Eating, in a short period of time, an amount of food that is definitely larger than most people would eat during a similar period of time and under similar circumstances • A feeling of lack of control over eating during the episode
Binge eating episodes accompanied by compensatory purging in order to prevent weight gain	• For example: self-induced vomiting; misuse of laxatives, diuretics, or other medications; fasting; or excessive exercise
Frequency	• Binge eating and compensatory behaviors occur at least once per week for 3 months
Sense of self	• Self-evaluation unduly influenced by body size or shape

uncomfortable swelling of the feet, to triggering rapid overall body weight increases, to accumulation of fluid in the lungs. What happens is that, in the context of chronic volume depletion, the body overproduces aldosterone in the adrenal glands. This hormone causes salt and water retention as well as urinary potassium losses. Pseudo-Bartter syndrome, as the secondary hyperaldosteronism is called, can be treated with purging cessation, slow rehydration, and several weeks of spironolactone, an aldosterone antagonist, under medical supervision.[29] While there are many other medical complications of purging, these are most important ones for practitioners to identify in order to refer their athletes to the proper specialists.

Resolution of Esteban's Case

Esteban receives appropriate care in the emergency department, assisted by his trainer advocating for him so that IV fluid is not given too quickly. He receives both IV and oral potassium replacement, and his EKG and lab values normalize. Esteban is ready for help. Ultimately, he wants to get back to a normal life and health. He is referred to a multidisciplinary team. It takes 4 months for his body weight and strength to recover, as he does emotional recovery work too. Esteban really wants to get back into his sport once he is in a better place. Given that wrestling carries a high focus on weight, his eating disorder team cautiously agrees, but will be keeping a close eye on him. His coach is counseled that Esteban clearly needs to compete in a higher weight class, given that he grew the summer before college started. The dietitian also respectfully lets the coach know that it is unscientific to recommend athletes eat "no more than 1 pound of food" on the night before a weigh-in, so they make weight. She underscores that 1 pound of food does not translate into 1 pound of body weight. Bodies break down food and use the calories for energy, and food weight in does not equate with body weight on the scale.

BINGE EATING

Case: Martin

Martin is a 21-year-old football player. Under pressure to make the starting lineup, he has been training harder than ever. He and his teammates agreed to go no-sugar for the season to make sure that their nutrition is optimized and their bodies are getting nothing but high protein and high calories. However, Martin has started bingeing on doughnuts late at night. He will eat a dozen behind closed doors, ravenously and rapidly devouring them. With his stomach uncomfortably full, he will go to bed, vowing that he will get back on track with his nutritional plans. He is so ashamed of not being able to keep up with the team's dietary plans that he tells no one. He has never purged. His weight starts to rise rapidly above his goal range.

Binge eating disorder is diagnosed by the DSM-V when a person has recurrent episodes of uncontrolled eating, associated with marked distress about the behavior, no purging, and 3 or more of the following criteria: eating rapidly; eating until uncomfortably full; eating large amounts of food when not hungry; eating alone due to embarrassment; or feeling disgusted, depressed, or guilty after a binge. The behaviors must occur at least once per week for 3 months for the formal diagnosis to be made. Binge eating disorder is the most common of the eating disorders, with a 2% to 4% population prevalence and equal representation of males and females (Table 4-3).

Many people inappropriately equate thinness with health. In reality, one cannot tell whether someone is healthy or unhealthy by looking at their size or shape. BMI (kg/m^2) is a poor measure of health, despite being used as a benchmark routinely. This is particularly true with athletes. Lauren might have had a BMI of 19 kg/m^2 as she descended into her AN, with multiple body systems malfunctioning, and yet have found herself squarely in the healthy range for BMI. Esteban would have also had a normal BMI while he was bingeing and purging, with critical electrolyte levels. Martin's teammates, who do not have binge eating disorder but have BMI levels in the "obese" range because of their muscularity, are some of the fittest young men in the country. Studies have shown that people in larger bodies with good exercise capacity live longer than those who rarely work out and are thin.[30] In addition, engaging in regular exercise yields life-prolonging benefits in multiple cardiovascular risk factors, independent of changes in body weight.[31]

TABLE 4-3	
BINGE EATING DIAGNOSTIC CRITERIA PER DSM-V	
CRITERION	DETAILS
Recurrent episodes of binge eating, without use of compensatory purging behaviors	• Eating, in a short period of time, an amount of food that is definitely larger than most people would eat during a similar period of time and under similar circumstances • A feeling of lack of control over eating during the episode
Binge eating episodes associated with 3 or more of the following	• Eating much more rapidly than normal • Eating until feeling uncomfortably full • Eating large amounts of food when not feeling physically hungry • Eating alone because of feeling embarrassed by how much one is eating • Feeling disgusted with oneself, depressed, or very guilty afterward
Emotional impact	• Binge eating episodes are markedly distressing
Frequency	• Binge eating occurs at least once per week for 3 months

Binge eating disorder is a full-fledged eating disorder. As such, Martin, too, requires referral to a multidisciplinary team with expertise in eating disorders. Probably the most important medical complication of binge eating disorder is poor overall care due to size stigma in the medical community. Martin, by virtue of being a football player and a male, risks not being identified and treated appropriately. Then, due to being in a larger body, he risks size stigma when he goes to the doctor. The **Health at Every Size** (HAES, pronounced "haze") philosophy is the gold standard for binge eating disorder treatment and really should be the gold standard for people of all sizes and shapes.[32] It encourages patients and clinicians to respect size diversity. It reminds us that eating enough food to nourish our bodies, without restrictions, and moving for joy and vitality, will most often result in our taking on the size and shape that were written in our genes. Eschewing a diet culture because diets have been proven over and over not to work, HAES urges people to ignore weight or weight loss as a primary target. Instead, it promotes a sustainable way of life. Even for elite athletes, HAES applies. One has only to look at top tennis players, swimmers, or any other sport to know that those who nourish themselves beautifully and practice their sport at the highest level still can look very different from each other in terms of size and shape.

Resolution of Martin's Case

Martin's practitioner has been keeping a close eye on him. Knowing Martin well, the practitioner notices that he has been acting more distant and that his weight has been rising rapidly. The practitioner knows how much it means to Martin to make the starting lineup. Finding a time when they have privacy, he asks Martin what is going on. Hearing about the team's resolution to eat no sugar, the practitioner identifies that this degree of restriction can set up cravings that lead to binges. In addition, intense stress or pressure, without possessing skills to ameliorate it, can intensify the risk of disordered eating. He lets Martin know his concerns that Martin has developed binge eating disorder and refers him to a multidisciplinary team. Martin may well be able to continue practicing during this work as he has no medical contraindications to participating in his sport. Ultimately, Martin and his team can collaborate to determine this.

CONCLUSION

Practitioners will serve their athletes best when they know about the different eating disorders and their main medical complications. Practitioners should never feel pressure to treat eating disorders. Rather, they have an obligation to their athletes never to promote pseudo-scientific associations between nutrition and performance, to recognize when an athlete is starting down the rabbit hole of disordered eating, and to refer appropriately to a multidisciplinary team with expertise in eating disorders when appropriate.

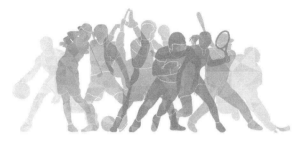

DEFINITIONS

Diagnostic and Statistical Manual of Mental Disorders (DSM-V): A model of describing mental disorders that offers a common language and standard criteria for the classification of mental disorders; it is used, or relied upon, by clinicians, researchers, psychiatric drug regulation agencies, and health insurance companies

DEXA bone density scan: Dual-energy x-ray absorptiometry (DEXA) or bone densitometry, is an enhanced form of x-ray technology that is used to measure bone loss; it can also be used to quantify body fat percentage in individuals

Health at Every Size: A social movement whose purpose is to encourage bodily acceptance and self-confidence with one's body, often by the rejection of dieting

REFERENCES

1. American Psychiatric Association. *Diagnostic and Statistical Manual of Mental Disorders: DSM-V.* Washington, DC: American Psychiatric Association; 2013.
2. Bratman S. The authorized Bratman orthorexia self-test. *Orthorexia.* http://www.orthorexia.com/. Accessed March 16, 2018.
3. Dunn TM, Bratman S. On orthorexia nervosa: a review of the literature and proposed diagnostic criteria. *Eat Behav.* 2016;21:11-17.
4. Moroze RM, Dunn TM, Holland JC, Yager J, Weintraub P. Microthinking about micronutrients: a case of transition from obsessions about healthy eating to near-fatal "orthorexia nervosa" and proposed diagnostic criteria. *Psychosomatics.* 2015;56(4):397-403.
5. Rosling AM, Sparén P, Norring C, von Knorring AL. Mortality of eating disorder: a follow-up study of treatment in a specialist unit 1974-2000. *Int J Eat Disord.* 2011;44(4):304-310.
6. Touyz S, Le Grange D, Lacey H, Hay P. *Managing Severe and Enduring Anorexia Nervosa.* New York, NY: Routledge; 2016.
7. Bombak AE, McPhail D, Ward P. Reproducing stigma: interpreting "overweight" and "obese" women's experiences of weight-based discrimination in reproductive healthcare. *Soc Sci Med.* 2016;166:94-101.
8. Phelan SM, Burgess DJ, Yeazel MW, Hellerstedt WL, Griffin JM, van Ryn M. Impact of weight bias and stigma on quality of care and outcomes for patients with obesity. *Obes Rev.* 2015;16(4):319-326.

9.   Martinsen M, Sundgot-Borgen J. Higher prevalence of eating disorders among adolescent elite athletes than controls. *Med Sci Sports Exerc.* 2013;45:1188-1197.

10.   Sundgot-Borgen J, Torstveit MK. Aspects of disordered eating continuum in elite high-intensity sports. *Scand J Med Sci Sports.* 2010;20(Suppl 2):112-121.

11.   Mountjoy M, Sundgot-Borgen J, Burke L, et al. The IOC consensus statement: beyond the Female Athlete Triad—Relative Energy Deficiency in Sport (RED-S). *Br J Sports Med.* 2014;48(7):491-497.

12.   Berner LA, Feig EH, Witt AA, Lowe MR. Menstrual cycle loss and resumption among patients with anorexia nervosa spectrum eating disorders: is relative or absolute weight more influential? *Int J Eat Disord.* 2017;50(4):442-446.

13.   Winkler LA, Frølich JS, Schulpen M, Støving RK. Body composition and menstrual status in adults with a history of anorexia nervosa-at what fat percentage is the menstrual cycle restored? *Int J Eat Disord.* 2017;50(4):370-377.

14.   Misra M, Golden NH, Katzman DK. State of the art systematic review of bone disease in anorexia nervosa. *Int J Eat Disord.* 2016;49(3):276-292.

15.   Faje AT, Fazeli PK, Miller KK, et al. Fracture risk and areal bone mineral density in adolescent females with anorexia nervosa. *Int J Eat Disord.* 2014;47(5):458-466.

16.   Olmos JM, Valero C, del Barrio AG, et al. Time course of bone loss in patients with anorexia nervosa. *Int J Eat Disord.* 2010;43(6):537-542.

17.   Gatti D, El Ghoch M, Viapiana O, et al. Strong relationship between vitamin D status and bone mineral density in anorexia nervosa. *Bone.* 2015;78:212-215.

18.   Misra M, Katzman D, Miller KK, et al. Physiologic estrogen replacement increases bone density in adolescent girls with anorexia nervosa. *J Bone Miner Res.* 2011;26:2430-2438.

19.   Southmayd EA, Hellmers AC, De Souza MJ. Food versus pharmacy: assessment of nutritional and pharmacological strategies to improve bone health in energy-deficient exercising women. *Curr Osteoporos Rep.* 2017;15(5):459-472.

20.   Baskaran C, Cunningham B, Plessow F, et al. Estrogen replacement improves verbal memory and executive control in oligomenorrheic/amenorrheic athletes in a randomized controlled trial. *J Clin Psychiatry.* 2017;78(5):e490-e497.

21.   Waugh EJ, Woodside DB, Beaton DE, Coté P, Hawker GA. Effects of exercise on bone mass in young women with anorexia nervosa. *Med Sci Sports Exerc.* 2011;43(5):755-763.

22.   Tenforde AS, Nattiv A, Ackerman K, Barrack MT, Fredericson M. Optimising bone health in the young male athlete. *Br J Sports Med.* 2017;51(3):148-149.

23.   Tenforde AS, Fredericson M, Sayres LC, et al. Identifying sex-specific risk factors for low bone mineral density in adolescent runners. *Am J Sports Med.* 2015;43:1494-1504.

24.   Barrack MT, Fredericson M, Tenforde AS, et al. Evidence of a cumulative effect for risk factors predicting lower bone mass among male adolescent athletes. *Br J Sports Med.* 2017;51:200-205.

25.   De Souza MJ, Nattiv A, Joy E, et al. 2014 Female Athlete Triad Coalition consensus statement on treatment and return to play of the female athlete triad: 1st International Conference held in San Francisco, CA, May 2012, and 2nd International Conference held in Indianapolis, IN, May 2013. *Clin J Sport Med.* 2014;24:96-119.

26.   Gaudiani JL, Sabel AL, Mascolo M, Mehler PS. Severe anorexia nervosa: outcomes from a medical stabilization unit. *Int J Eat Disord.* 2012;45(1):85-92.

27.   Sabel AL, Gaudiani JL, Statland B, Mehler PS. Hematologic abnormalities in severe anorexia nervosa. *Ann Hematol.* 2013;92(5):605-613.

28.   Rosen E, Sabel AL, Brinton JT, Catanach B, Gaudiani JL, Mehler PS. Liver dysfunction in patients with severe anorexia nervosa. *Int J Eat Disord.* 2016;49(2):151-158.

29. Bahia A, Mascolo M, Gaudiani JL, Mehler PS. Pseudobartter syndrome in eating disorders. *Int J Eat Disord.* 2012;45(1):150-153.

30. Lavie CJ, De Schutter A, Milani RV. Healthy obese versus unhealthy lean: the obesity paradox. *Nat Rev Endocrinol.* 2015;11(1):55-62.

31. Italian Diabetes Exercise Study (IDES) Investigators; Balducci S, Zanuso S, Cardelli P, et al. Changes in physical fitness predict improvements in modifiable cardiovascular risk factors independently of body weight loss in subjects with type 2 diabetes participating in the Italian Diabetes and Exercise Study (IDES). *Diabetes Care.* 2012;35(6):1347-1354.

32. Bacon L. *Health at Every Size.* https://haescommunity.com/. Retrieved March 16, 2018.

Open any exercise physiology textbook and the first factor of importance to fatigue is a reduction of blood volume with its associated hormonal responses, with the second, less impressive, factor being decreased carbohydrate availability. Why? Simplistically, you can fix low circulating carbohydrate pretty effectively by eating something and feeling the effects within minutes. A reduction in blood volume is more complex, taking hours to rectify and involving a series of hormonal and electrochemical gradient feedback mechanisms.

Blood volume is a combination of the red blood cells and plasma in circulation. When discussing exercise and fluid shifts, the term *plasma volume* is often used, as this refers to the watery component of blood. As you continue exercise, a competition exists as the muscles and skin fight for circulating blood. Blood goes to the muscles for metabolic function. Blood goes to the skin to get rid of the heat produced by the working muscles. As body water drops, this competition becomes fiercer. As exercise continues and plasma volume is lost through sweating, breathing, and gastrointestinal water usage, available circulating blood diminishes; there is less overall water in the blood, thus it is "thicker."

This redistribution cannot continue indefinitely as the demands of exercise and thermoregulation will exceed the cardiovascular system's ability to meet these demands. Ultimately, blood distribution to the skin will decrease in favor of delivery to the exercising muscles, increasing thermal stress and eventually risking heat illness. When the body reaches this point, it becomes unable to keep the status quo against the rising temperature of the muscles and overall core temperature. These temperature points usually signal the body to cease exercise. The first aspect of fatigue is the tipping point of muscle temperature over 102°F, at which point the contractile proteins start to physically break down. The second point is core temperature reaching ~104°F to 105.8°F (40°C to 41°C), signaling changes to the central nervous system to slow down or cease exercise. Note here that it is not just the core temperature that dictates performance impairment, but the overall thermal stress and decreased blood availability. The most trying situation for the body is the combination of hot skin, low body water, and elevated core temperature. During exercise, the most stressful physiological burden is support of high skin blood flow made worse by exercising in the heat. Skin temperature is affected more so by ambient temperature; core temperature is affected by exercise intensity and is largely independent from environmental factors when heat can be offloaded effectively through the body's thermoregulatory system. With hot skin, there is less cooling available to return to the body and low body water impacts blood volume, reducing sweat capacity and the body's ability to offload heat. This situation will increase heat stress, increase heat storage, and thus increase physiologic strain.[1,2] The point of contention, however, is at what percent body mass loss does performance decline occur?

What IS Hydration?
The Physiology of Fluid Absorption

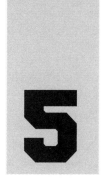

Stacy Sims, BSc, MSc, PhD

Key Takeaways

* There are many aspects that affect hydration such as body temperature, air temperature, type and intensity of exercise, and other facets that should be considered.
* Dehydration has been extolled as the limiting factor to both the anaerobic and aerobic components of exercise.
* Research has indicated that in elite athletes (highly trained individuals), mild to moderate loss of body water (>3% body mass loss) has minimal to no effect on performance in cool and neutral condition, and can handle more moderate temperatures with performance loss.
* A winning sports drink is composed of significantly less sugar than most brand name sports drinks currently on the market.
* Ideal sports drinks for fluid absorption (aka a functional hydration beverage) should contain 3% to 4% carbohydrate (from glucose and sucrose) with sodium and potassium.

Amato D. *An Athletic Trainer's Guide to Sports Nutrition (pp 65-76).*
© 2019 SLACK Incorporated.

PERFORMANCE, HEAT STRESS, AND BODY WATER

Thermoregulation and Body Fluids

Besides vasodilation, evaporative heat loss through sweating is the other primary defense against heat storage in the body. The loss of body fluids through sweating leads to dehydration, threatening fluid balance and further challenging blood redistribution to the muscles and skin.[3] Physical activity increases total metabolic rate to provide energy for skeletal muscle contraction, and 70% to almost 100% of this metabolically generated heat needs to be dissipated. Depending on environmental humidity and temperature, the hotter the environment, the greater the dependence on evaporative heat loss via sweating.[4] A reduction of the central circulating blood volume due to either reduced blood volume (hypovolemia) accompanying dehydration, or the dilation of the peripheral blood vessels, results in a fall in the cardiac filling pressure and stroke volume. If left uncompensated, cardiac output will be compromised.

Hypohydration—the sustained state of low fluid balance—inhibits thermoregulatory responses to heat stress, and both **hypovolemia** and plasma hyperosmolality (increased electrolyte concentration) impairs thermoregulatory responses such as vasodilation and sweating.[5] At the onset of acute heat stress, even before any reduction in total body water through sweating, shifts in body fluid occur between the bloodstream and the surrounding tissue spaces due to blood pressure changes. With sweating, a reduction of total body water occurs in particular if adequate amounts of fluid are not consumed. Hypohydration affects the water content in each of the compartments. The initial body water loss mostly comes from the blood volume and fluid in between the cells. However, as body water loss increases, a proportionately greater percentage of water deficit comes from within the cells themselves.[6] Water appears to be lost from the plasma at a rate 1 to 5 times that of other fluid compartments, with relatively greater plasma water loss accompanied by sodium ions lost through sweat and urine. Nose and colleagues[7] investigated the relationship between sodium [Na^+] in sweat and the distribution of body water during dehydrating exercise. A linear relationship exists between the change of extracellular fluid and the change in plasma volume, indicating that it is the increase in plasma concentration that shifts fluid from the intracellular to the extracellular compartments to maintain plasma volume.

The amounts of electrolytes lost in sweat are typically reduced with heat acclimation as the sodium and chloride lost with sweat are primarily from the extracellular compartment. It has been reported that, over the course of heat acclimation, the sweat sodium concentration decreases by ~59% despite an increase of sweat rate by 12%.[8] Hence, for a given sweat rate in heat-acclimated individuals, the solute lost from the plasma is significantly reduced, allowing for a greater shift of fluid from the intracellular to extracellular compartments, which would lessen the loss of blood volume compared to an unacclimated individual.

Historically, dehydration has been extolled as the limiting factor to both the anaerobic and aerobic components of exercise. The longstanding view has been that critical levels of water deficit exist at which exercise performance is impaired. Early studies indicated that small (2%) to moderate (4%) body mass loss impacts oxygen uptake in a hot environment[9] along with heart rate and core temperature.[10] It was traditionally thought that the primary factor of fatigue was due to a drop in body water, critical for thermoregulation and muscle blood flow; however, hypohydration can increase several forms of physiological stress during physical activity, including metabolic (glycogen depletion), thermal, oxidative, and immune. Furthermore, laboratory studies attenuate the vast role of psychological and physiological behavior due to the tightly controlled study environment(s). It is well-known that increased psychophysical strain is directly proportional to increased physiological strain, which, in turn, drives behavior.[11]

To examine the prevailing theory that the interaction of skin temperature, core temperature, and hypohydration have adverse effects on exercise performance, several investigators examined the effect of high skin vs high core temperature with and without dehydration on exercise performance. Cheuvront et al[12] tested the effect of hypohydration on aerobic performance utilizing a protocol of 30 minutes of exercise at ~50% VO_{2peak}, followed by a 30-minute time trial (TT) in temperate and cold environments. A small 3% body mass loss (5% body water loss) impaired performance by 8% in the temperate (T_{sk} ~29°C), but not in the cold environment (T_{sk} ~20°C). Castellani et al[13] employed a similar protocol of a preload exercise at a set intensity followed by a TT, with a T_{sk} of ~32°C in both hypohydration and euhydration trials. With warm skin, a 4% body mass loss impaired performance by 18% as compared to the warm skin with euhydration with no significant differences in core temperature across trials. Kenefick et al[14] further tested the interaction between environmental conditions and hypohydration by having participants cycle for 30 minutes (50% VO_{2peak}) followed by a 15-minute TT in 10°C, 20°C, 30°C, and 40°C environments (inducing stepwise increases in T_{sk} from 26°C to 36°C) when euhydrated and when hypohydrated by 4% body mass. Core temperature did not differ across the hypo- and euhydration trials; hypohydration impaired aerobic performance by 12% and 23% when T_{sk} was 33°C and 36°C, respectively. Collectively, these studies demonstrated that hypohydration degrades aerobic performance to a greater extent with increasing heat stress; yet it is critical to note that none of these studies considered the factors differentiating the effects of hypohydration in a lab vs autonomous outdoor exercise (among which include thirst/drive to drink, training status, airflow speed, blinding to hydration status, familiarization to the stress of the experimental trials, exercise pacing, and motivation to perform).

Thirst plays a significant role in fluid balance (as it is one of the key psychologic factors to replace lost fluid), and can influence motivation as well as performance outcomes. For example, thirst can trigger decreased exercise intensity to prevent further fluid loss. In studies of dehydration, water is deliberately withheld to induce hypohydration; however, when exercise-induced body mass loss to 2% to 3% is achieved voluntarily by drinking *ad libitum*, no measurable effect on exercise performance has been determined in trained individuals.[15] When using realistic airflow in temperate conditions with *ad libitum* drinking, no effects of 2.5% hypohydration were found in trained cyclists over an 80-minute exercise trial, whereas indications of greater thermal strain and performance power decline was found in untrained cyclists.[16] Moreover, Mora-Rodriguez and colleagues[17] determined that fluid ingestion reduced thermal and cardiovascular strain in unacclimated and trained, but not untrained, cyclists during moderate exercise in the heat.

Recently, Cheung and colleagues[18] conducted a seminal study to determine the effects of thirst and dehydration on cycling performance in the heat. Participants were trained and acclimated to exercise in the heat and familiarized to the experimental sessions to reduce cofounding psychological variables. The study employed either blinded sham or real IV infusion for hydration control, with simultaneous thirst manipulation through the use of water mouth rinse or no rinse. This allowed 4 conditions to be tested: dehydrated with and without thirst sensation and euhydrated with and without thirst sensation. Importantly, the participants had no clues to their actual hydration status because of the IV blinding. The final outcomes indicated that greater thermal strain occurred in the dehydrated conditions during the 20-km self-paced TT, but no performance metric (power output, 20 km TT completion times, pacing profiles) were affected by either moderate dehydration (> 2% to 3% body mass loss) and thirst.

What Is the Takeaway?

Recent research has indicated that, in elite athletes (highly trained individuals), mild to moderate loss of body water (> 3% body mass loss) has minimal to no effect on performance in cool and neutral conditions. In warm to hot conditions, these athletes can tolerate the conditions of low body water (up to 6% body mass loss) without suffering heat illness, although there is a decrease in performance (in particular, endurance performance).[19] However, in less-trained athletes (eg, recreational, new to sport, return to training after > 6 months off), mild to moderate hypohydration does have an impact on exercise performance,[17] but you must also consider the psychological aspects of self-pacing, thirst sensation, discomfort of exercise, and heat, which all may play a significant role in motivation. Additional research should be done to examine the effects of greater dehydration (> 5% body mass loss) on fluid balance hormones, sex differences, pacing, and autonomous outdoor exercise performance to determine the true effect of fluid intake on realistic performance measures.

BLOOD VOLUME AND FLUID ABSORPTION

If blood volume drops (due to loss of water), what impact does this have on nutrient uptake and how does this affect performance? The intestine is the primary organ for absorption of fluids, nutrients, and electrolytes. During prolonged exercise that increases core temperature, blood flow to the gastrointestinal (GI) tract may be reduced by up to 80% to provide sufficient blood to the working muscles and skin. As core temperature approaches 39°C, the intestinal temperature may be as high as 41°C, leading to cell damage. In addition, the shunting of blood away from the intestines causes ischemia and oxidative damage. Both results can compromise the integrity of the intestinal tract, from large-action motility to the small action of epithelial cell tight junction permeability. The disruption to the tight junction proteins results in an increased release of luminal **endotoxins** (also known as *intestinal bacteria*) into the blood stream. These endotoxins increase systemic immune response, inflammation, and oxidation and perpetuate GI dysfunction.

As an athlete, you should be concerned with how to mitigate this drop in blood volume and reduced blood flow to the GI system. What you eat and drink plays a critical part on your overall performance by delaying fatigue or maintaining power due to their effects on fluid dynamics.

The main factors that affect fluid absorption include the following:

* The composition of what you are drinking, such as osmolality, carb choices, and sodium content
* Gastric emptying, or how fast a solution exits the stomach and enters the small intestines)
* Hypo- vs hyperosmotic changes in the intestinal lumen
* Co-transport mechanisms

Let us look at the key factors needed to pull fluid into the body's fluid spaces. Ninety-five percent of all fluid absorption occurs in the small intestines, and this organ is very particular to osmotic and electrochemical gradients. Moreover, when you start to exercise, 60% to 80% of your blood is diverted away from the gut to meet the muscle and skin demands for blood. With this, you need to drink something that works with your physiology.

The normal osmolality of the intestinal lumen of a fasted individual sits between 270 and 290 mosmol/kg, or isotonic with respect to blood. When food or fluid is consumed, the osmolality changes with accordance to the rate at which the nutrients are emptied from the stomach into the small intestines. However, the proximal small intestines (duodenum and upper jejunum) are very particular to osmotic and electrochemical gradients; thus, returning to **isotonicity** becomes the priority. The time it takes to achieve isotonicity varies with what has been consumed, and thus the composition of the solution is critical for rapid fluid absorption.

Hypertonic solutions (eg, solutions with an osmolality ≥ 290 mosmol/kg) cause a net movement of water from circulation into the intestinal lumen to dilute the contents. The greater the initial osmolality, the greater the rate of water efflux due to the greater osmotic gradient between the contents of the lumen and the intestinal cells. Moreover, the time lapse for achieving isotonicity increases the contact time of the solution with the intestinal walls, rendering hyperosmotic solutions ineffective in promoting hydration (Figure 5-1).

To further complicate the issue, plain water is associated with a poor rate of water absorption, primarily due to the outward flow of sodium down electrochemical gradients, pulling both water and sodium into the lumen.

Studies have shown that solutions containing carbs and sodium, but maintaining an osmolality less than 200 mosmol/kg, achieve slower rates of water absorption than solutions of an osmolality between ~200 to 260 mosmol/kg. Although this is a tight range of osmolality, even the smallest differences can have significant effects on fluid

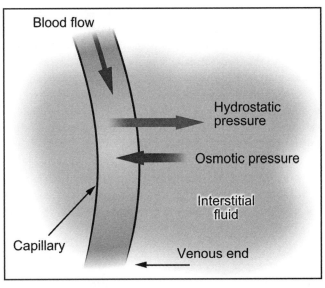

absorption. For example, the comparison of 3 solutions composed of glucose and sodium but with different osmolalities illustrates this point succinctly. A hypotonic solution (229 mosmol/kg) produced twice as rapid net water absorption into the bloodstream as compared to the isotonic (277 mosmol/kg), with again significantly less water absorption with the hypertonic (352 mosmol/kg) solution. Moreover, an increased rate of glucose absorption is associated with the faster water absorption rates of the hypotonic solution but no difference of solute absorption between the isotonic and hypertonic solutions.[20] Further studies tested the effect of osmolality on fluid absorption. Trends for faster fluid absorption and directionally greater relative plasma volume were observed in solutions of lower osmolality for the same absolute carb content or lower carb (2% vs 6%) ingested,[21] respectively.

When we examine the carb used in solutions, points of contention are apparent. The sodium-glucose co-transport mechanism is critical for both fluid and glucose absorption across the cell membranes, and these are interlinked rather than separate pathways. Glucose is absorbed by the small intestine using an active process. Initially, the glucose and fluid exits the intestinal lumen via the sodium-glucose co-transporter proteins (SGLT-1 and SGLT-5), and is facilitated through an additional protein "gate" of GLUT-2. With the glucose, water and sodium also enter the blood, contributing to blood volume. When fructose and glucose are ingested in combination (either as fructose plus glucose, or as sucrose) the mean oxidized amount of the mixed sugars is ~66%, as opposed to fructose at 29% (women) to 45% (men) and glucose at 58%.

The actual absorption rate of the sugars is the contention here: glucose is absorbed from the intestine into the plasma via more than one active glucose co-transporter protein, reducing the contact time with the gut lumen. Fructose, however, is less efficient and slower to be absorbed due to less active transport mechanisms, leading to increased contact time with the gut lumen. Why is contact time significant? With incomplete and slow absorption, fructose produces a hyperosmolar environment in the intestines. What this means is that there is more solute than water, causing an increased osmotic pressure. This in turn signals fluid to be drawn into the intestines, producing the common feelings of bloating, gas, diarrhea, and general GI discomfort.

Maltodextrin, a polysaccharide with the building blocks of glucose, is used in many sports drinks instead of straight glucose for several reasons. The primary rationale is that maltodextrin does not affect osmolality as significantly as glucose, fructose, or dextrose. Because maltodextrin is a long chain of glucose molecules, it does not add as much to the number of solutes in a solution, thus a solution can contain quite a bit of maltodextrin and still have a faster gastric emptying rate. From a carb availability standpoint, this is appealing because glucose molecules are absorbed through the several glucose co-transporter proteins. Here is the caveat: although a maltodextrin solution can be hypotonic—which, in theory, should promote water absorption—the hydrolysis of maltodextrin elevates luminal osmolality, creating the same hyperosmolar environment in the intestines as fructose and slowing the rate of water absorption.

A single beverage suitable for all environmental and race conditions probably does not exist. To maximize water absorption, consideration should be given to beverages formulated with 1) glucose and sucrose (to enhance fluid uptake via co-transport mechanisms) in concentrations of 2% to 4% to reduce osmolality; and 2) sodium to reduce sodium secretion in the duodenum, which serves to attenuate the osmotic flow of water from the blood into the intestinal lumen.

THE WINNING (AND NOT WINNING) SOLUTION

What is the winning solution for hydration? It is not the ones so many recreational (and even professional) athletes use. Here are the nutritional aspects of a typical non-winning, carb-heavy sports drink per 8 ounces:

* 5% to 8% carb solution (12 to 19 g carb)
* Osmolality of around 300 to 305 mosmol/kg
* Sugars: maltodextrin, fructose, sucrose
* Sodium: 52 to 110 mg
* Examples include Gatorade (PepsiCo), Powerade and VitaminWater (Coca Cola Company), PowerBar (Premier Nutrition Corporation), Tailwind (Tailwind Nutrition), UCAN (The UCAN Company), Cytomax (Cytosport), HEED and Perpetuum (Hammer Nutrition), and Electrolyte Hydrator (Vega Sport).

Instead, you want to seek out a sports drink that supplies some glucose, sodium, and other key co-transporters as described previously. A winning solution contains the following per 8 ounces:

* 3% to 4% carb solution (7 to 9.4 g carb)
* Sugars: 7 to 9.4 g from glucose and sucrose
* Sodium: 180 to 225 mg
* Potassium: 60 to 75 mg (another fluid co-transporter that can help sodium)
* Examples include NUUN Performance (Nuun & Company, Inc), Osmo Hydration (Osmo Nutrition), Clif Shot Hydration electrolyte drink (Clif Bar & Company), Hydration Drink Mix (GU Energy Labs).

EXERCISE-ASSOCIATED HYPONATREMIA AND SEX DIFFERENCES

Critical to maintaining **extracellular fluid volume** (ECFV) is sodium. When sweating takes place without fluid replacement, total body water is reduced from each fluid compartment due to the free exchange of water between compartments with a concomitant loss of electrolytes, primarily sodium. When plasma volume loss is due to total body water loss, the kidneys also act to retain sodium and water to restore total ECFV. As sodium and other electrolytes do not act as effective vascular osmotic agents because they freely diffuse across capillary endothelium, changes in sodium content are related to the changes in total ECFV.[22] Therefore, the balance of sodium in the body is crucial to maintain ECFV. Commercially available sports drinks typically contain 10 to 20 mmol $Na^+ \cdot L^{-1}$ (20 to 40 mmol L^{-1} Na^+; 3 to 15 mmol L^{-1} K+, 6% CHO [roughly 12 to 19 g of carbs with about 52 to 110 mg of sodium per 8 oz]), which research has shown to be less than adequate for sodium restoration during dehydration from prolonged exercise or heat stress.[23]

Exercise-associated hyponatremia (EAH), sometimes called *water intoxication*, refers to reductions in the body's sodium level during or up to 24 hours after physical activity; hyponatremia occurs from a dilution of the extracellular fluid with or without an excess of body water volume.

Women are at greater risk for exercise-induced hyponatremia (low blood sodium concentration), and this risk has been attributed to their lower body weight and size, excess water ingestion, and longer racing times relative to men. While these factors contribute to the greater incidence of hyponatremia in women, it is likely that their greater levels of estradiol in plasma and/or tissue also play a role in increasing the risk of hyponatremia in women.[24] The basic physiology of sodium and fluid dynamics is well understood. However, plasma volume in women is highly influenced by estrogen and progesterone. Estrogen and progesterone can have profound effects on fluid dynamics, in particular the Starling forces that regulate fluid movement between the vascular and interstitial spaces altering plasma volume (Figure 5-2).[25]

The hormonal influences of the menstrual cycle affect fluid dynamics by altering capillary permeability, vasomotor function, and the central set-point control of renal

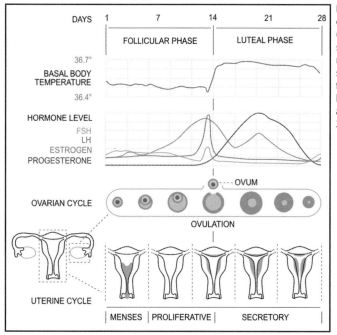

Figure 5-2. The endogenous menstrual cycle. (Reprinted with permission from Physiological responses to the menstrual cycle: implications for the development of heat illness in female athletes. *Sports Med.* 2002;32:601-614.)

hormones and plasma osmolality.[26] The elevations in plasma progesterone concentrations during the luteal phase inhibit aldosterone-dependent sodium reabsorption at the kidneys due to progesterone competing with aldosterone for the mineralocorticoid receptor; thus, there is an increase in total body sodium excretion. For example, Stachenfeld et al[27] have observed that the mean concentrations of aldosterone and plasma renin activity are greater in the mid-luteal phase than in the follicular phase. Thus, with a reduction of aldosterone-dependent sodium reabsorption, a phase-dependent increase in sodium excretion occurs. With this increased excretion, the body responds by stimulating the renin–angiotensin–aldosterone system to try to hold on to additional sodium in the luteal phase. However, this competition results in little, if any, overall water retention but does induce fluid shifts away from the plasma, reducing plasma volume by ~8% in the luteal phase.

With these hormonal influences and physiologic perturbations in fluid balance, the signal for thirst—driven by plasma osmolality and, to some extent, volume with the transient hypovolemia—is dampened; the set point of osmolality is lower and women are hypovolemic as compared to the low hormone phase. Thirst sensitivity is lessened as a physiological construct, otherwise women would go crazy with the drive to drink in the high hormone phase, yet they are closer to the clinical definition of hyponatremia in the luteal phase due to the aforementioned physiological changes.

Summary

The complexity of the body extends well into the aspect of "hydration" and what it means to maintain body fluids for health and for performance. The following guidelines may help:

* Drink to thirst during exercise if:
  ○ You have prehydrated prior to the training session or race; otherwise, dehydration can predispose you to tissue injury, decreased motivation during exercise, and poor recovery (adaptations, sleep, rehydration).
  ○ You are heat acclimated.
  ○ You are adequately trained (after significant time off with lower fitness levels, dehydration and exercise stress can exacerbate thermal strain and decrease your performance metrics).
  ○ You have a history of EAH or have syndrome of inappropriate antidiuretic hormone secretion.
* Drink on a schedule during exercise if:
  ○ You are a junior athlete and have not gone through puberty.
  ○ You have 2 or more heavy training sessions in a day to avoid systemic dehydration.
  ○ You are not acclimated and training at altitude.
  ○ You have a history of heat illness.

Conclusion

* The goal of hydration is to keep your body fluid levels high enough to get rid of the heat you produce and cool you down while you are exercising.
* Separate your fueling from your hydration.
* Do not depend on a typical sports drink for hydration. These sports drinks are about 5% to 8% carb with a low level of sodium and other key electrolytes. This carb concentration provides some energy for exercise, but it comes at the expense of hydration because it is too high to maximize fluid absorption in your gut.
* An ideal sports drink for fluid absorption (ie, a functional hydration beverage) should contain 3% to 4% carb (from glucose and sucrose) with sodium and potassium.
* You are more predisposed to hyponatremia (water intoxication) during the luteal (high-hormone) phase of your menstrual cycle.

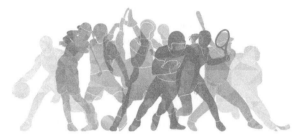

DEFINITIONS

Hypovolemia: A decreased volume of blood circulating in the body

Endotoxins: A heat-stable toxin associated with the outer membranes of certain gram-negative bacteria, released when cells are disrupted

Isotonicity: Possessing and maintaining a uniform tone or tension

Extracellular fluid volume: Bodily fluid outside of cells

Exercise-associated hyponatremia: A fluid-electrolyte disorder caused by a decrease in sodium levels after prolonged physical activity

REFERENCES

1. Gagge AP, Stolwijk JA, Hardy JD. Comfort and thermal sensations and associated physiological responses at various ambient temperatures. *Environ Res.* 1967;1:1-20.
2. Sawka MN, Cheuvront SN, Kenefick RW. High skin temperature and hypohydration impair aerobic performance. *Exp Physiol.* 2012;97:327-332.
3. Armstrong LE, Maresh CM. Effects of training, environment, and host factors on the sweating response to exercise. *Int J Sports Med.* 1998;19(Suppl 2):S103-S15.
4. Sawka MN, Gonzalez RR, Young AJ, Dennis RC, Valeri CR, Pandolf KB. Control of thermoregulatory sweating during exercise in the heat. *Am J Physiol.* 1989;257:R311-R316.
5. Cheuvront SN, Kenefick RW. Dehydration: physiology, assessment, and performance effects. *Compr Physiol.* 2014;4(1):257-285.
6. Costill DL, Cote R, Fink W. Muscle water and electrolytes following varied levels of dehydration in man. *J Appl Physiol.* 1976;40:6-11.
7. Nose H, Mack GW, Shi X, Nadel ER. Involvement of sodium retention hormones during rehydration in humans. *J Appl Physiol.* 1988;65:332-336.
8. Kirby CR, Convertino VA. Plasma aldosterone and sweat sodium concentrations after exercise and heat acclimation. *J Appl Physiol.* 1986;61:967-970.
9. Sawka MN. Physiological consequences of hypohydration: exercise performance and thermoregulation. *Med Sci Sports Exerc.* 1992;24:657-670.
10. Montain SJ, Coyle EF. Influence of graded dehydration on hyperthermia and cardiovascular drift during exercise. *J Appl Physiol.* 1992;73:1340-1350.

11. Tucker R. The anticipatory regulation of performance: the physiological basis for pacing strategies and the development of a perception-based model for exercise performance. *Br J Sports Med.* 2009;43:392-400.

12. Cheuvront SN, Carter R 3rd, Castellani JW, Sawka MN. Hypohydration impairs endurance exercise performance in temperate but not cold air. *J Appl Physiol.* 2005;99:1972-1976.

13. Castellani JW, Muza SR, Cheuvront SN, et al. Effect of hypohydration and altitude exposure on aerobic exercise performance and acute mountain sickness. *J Appl Physiol.* 2010;109:1792-1800.

14. Kenefick RW, Cheuvront SN, Palombo LJ, Ely BR, Sawka MN. Skin temperature modifies the impact of hypohydration on aerobic performance. *J Appl Physiol.* 2010;109:79-86.

15. Goulet EDB. Effect of exercise-induced dehydration on time-trial exercise performance: a meta-analysis. *Br J Sports Med.* 2011;45:1149-1156.

16. Merry TL, Ainslie PN, Cotter JD. Effects of aerobic fitness on hypohydration-induced physiological strain and exercise impairment. *Acta Physiol (Oxf).* 2010;198:179-190.

17. Mora-Rodriguez R, Hamouti N, Del Coso J, Ortega JF. Fluid ingestion is more effective in preventing hyperthermia in aerobically trained than untrained individuals during exercise in the heat. *Appl Physiol Nutr Metab.* 2013;38:73-80.

18. Cheung SS, McGarr GW, Mallette MM, et al. Separate and combined effects of dehydration and thirst sensation on exercise performance in the heat. *Scand J Med Sci Sports.* 2015;25(Suppl 1):104-111.

19. Beis LY, Wright-Whyte M, Fudge B, Noakes T, Pitsiladis YP. Drinking behaviors of elite male runners during marathon competition. *Clin J Sport Med.* 2012;22:254-261.

20. Gisolfi CV, Summers RD, Schedl HP, Bleiler TL. Effect of sodium concentration in a carbohydrate-electrolyte solution on intestinal absorption. *Med Sci Sports Exerc.* 1995;27:1414-1420.

21. Rogers J, Summers RW, Lambert GP. Gastric emptying and intestinal absorption of a low-carbohydrate sport drink during exercise. *Int J Sport Nutr Exerc Metab.* 2005;15:220-235.

22. Harrison MH. Effects of thermal stress and exercise on blood volume in humans. *Physiol Rev.* 1985;65:149-208.

23. Vrijens DM, Rehrer NJ. Sodium-free fluid ingestion decreases plasma sodium during exercise in the heat. *J Appl Physiol.* 1999;86:1847-1851.

24. Hew-Butler T, Rosner MH, Fowkes-Godek S, et al. Statement of the Third International Exercise-Associated Hyponatremia Consensus Development Conference, Carlsbad, California, 2015. *Clin J Sport Med.* 2015;25:303-320.

25. Marsh SA, Jenkins DG. Physiological responses to the menstrual cycle: implications for the development of heat illness in female athletes. *Sports Med.* 2002;32:601-614.

26. Oian P, Tollan A, Fadnes HO, Noddeland H, Maltau JM. Transcapillary fluid dynamics during the menstrual cycle. *Am J Obstet Gynecol.* 1987;156:952-955.

27. Stachenfeld NS, DiPietro L, Kokoszka CA, Silva C, Keefe DL, Nadel ER. Physiological variability of fluid-regulation hormones in young women. *J Appl Physiol.* 1999;86(3):1092-1096.

It can be quite daunting trying to keep up with all of the supplements that come out seemingly on a daily basis for almost any malady. Many are harmless and, in some cases, do not even contain the supplement advertised on the bottle. There are some independent regulatory agencies that test supplements and provide results for a fee, but it would be impossible for them to keep up with the overwhelming number of supplement companies that are not regulated in the United States. The landmark Dietary Supplement Health and Education Act of 1994 (DSHEA) is a statute of United States Federal legislation that defines and regulates dietary supplements.[1] The act defined supplements and effectively regulated them by FDA enforcement for Good Manufacturing Practices under 21 CFR Part 111.[2] The act essentially deregulated the entire supplement industry, prompting an explosion of companies making absurd claims about myriad different supplements, with no one to tell them their claims were at best a waste of money, and at worst incredibly dangerous to the consumer of the product. Luckily, a quick internet search on a smart phone can assist a practitioner in looking up almost everything he or she might need to know about a supplement that an athlete may ask about.

While practitioners should educate themselves on the more common supplements that athletes take, the entirety of that is beyond the scope of this text. The most common supplements taken will be the focus, that being protein, creatine, and caffeine. Not only are these the most common supplements that athletes take, they are also the most well researched. Even so, arguments still arise among nutrition professionals regarding the use, dosage, and efficacy of each.

Supplements

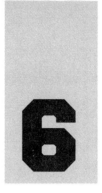

KEY TAKEAWAYS

* There are an innumerable amount of athletic performance-enhancing supplements on the market, but practitioners would do well to be very educated on the most common, such as creatine, caffeine, and protein.
* There are multiple aspects of animal protein that make it a higher quality source in relation to plant proteins.
* Overall protein intake for athletes is a widely debated topic that still warrants further research and should be handled on an individual basis.
* While creatine is the most heavily researched supplement available, there are still gaps in the research to appropriately prescribe type, dosage, and frequency.
* Many supplement claims are not backed by proper research and should not be taken with proper monitoring by educated practitioners.

PROTEIN

Structure

Proteins are composed of amino acids. It has many functions including structural components of cells, contractile filaments, antibodies for human responses, transporters, neurotransmitters, hormones, and enzymes. There are over 140 amino

Amato D. *An Athletic Trainer's Guide to Sports Nutrition (pp 79-111).* © 2019 SLACK Incorporated.

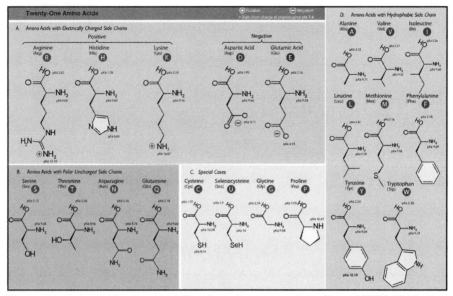

Figure 6-1. Amino acids. (Reprinted from https://commons.wikimedia.org/wiki/File%3AAmino_Acids-wide.svg. By Bert Hubert [CC BY-SA 4.0 (https://creativecommons.org/licenses/by-sa/4.0)], via Wikimedia Commons from Wikimedia Commons.)

acid types known; however, our body generally only uses 20 of them. Amino acids are linked together by peptide bonds. There are 3 different classifications of amino acids: an aliphatic amino acid has straight carbon chains, an aromatic amino acid has ring structures, and acidic and basic amino acids are classified on their pH within an aqueous solution (Figure 6-1).

There are 8 to 9 amino acids that are considered essential as human cells are unable to adequately synthesize them to meet the needs for growth and maintenance. These essential amino acids are lysine, tryptophan, methionine, valine, phenylalanine, leucine, isoleucine, and threonine. Histidine is an essential amino acid in infants. Methionine and phenylalanine can be converted to cysteine and tyrosine, but if these are inadequate in the diet or other conditions inhibit conversion, these 2 amino acids also become essential. An amino acid can be referred to as a *limiting amino acid* if one of the essential amino acids present in a food is in an amount insufficient to support growth or maintenance. All essential amino acids must be present and in the right quantity in order to make protein; if even one amino acid is not at appropriate levels, the whole system ceases to work.

Function

* Hormones: Many hormones are created by and in fact are proteins. These hormones assist in controlling body functions, especially those functions that involve organs. Insulin, for example, is a hormone that regulates blood sugar. It involves the interaction of organs such as the pancreas and liver. It is well-known

that insulin facilitates the activation of the **mammalian target of rapamycin (mTOR) pathway**, particularly high insulin levels. Leucine is a direct activator of the mTOR pathway and is able to "switch on" protein synthesis in muscle cells.

* Transporting and storing particles: Protein is paramount in transportation of certain molecules. Hemoglobin, for example, is a protein that transports oxygen throughout the body. Ferritin is a protein that combines with iron for storage in the liver. Both are vital functions of protein in the body.

* Antibodies: Antibodies are formed by protein to prevent infections and diseases. These specific proteins identify and assist in destroying antigens such as bacteria and viruses. They often work in combination with the other immune system cells such a T-cells. These antibodies identify and then surround antigens in order to keep them contained until they can be destroyed by white blood cells.

* Restoration and preservation: Protein is often referred to as the "building blocks of the body." That may be an oversimplification, however, because protein is dynamic in the maintenance of body tissue, including development and repair. Hair, nails, skin, muscles, and organs are all made from protein. This is why children need more protein per pound of body weight than adults; they are growing and developing new protein tissue and require more protein to increase the size of not only their muscular and bone tissue, but that of organ tissue as well.

* Enzymes: Enzymes are proteins that change the rate of chemical reactions in the body. In fact, most of the necessary chemical reactions in the body would not efficiently proceed without enzymes. One type of enzyme functions as an aid in digesting large protein, carbohydrate, and fat molecules into smaller molecules, while another assists the creation of DNA. Salivary amylase, found primarily in saliva and pancreatic fluid, converts starch and glycogen into simple sugars.

* Energy: Protein is a minor source of energy. If you consume more protein than you need for body tissue maintenance and other essential functions, your body will use it for energy, especially if you eat too little fat. The human body can do 3 things with protein calories: put protein in fat stores, use it as an energy source, or use it to carry out functions vital to life. Protein calories will be used as an energy source when the body is lacking fat or carb calories for fuel. When the body receives sufficient quantities of proteins, fats, and carbs, protein will carry out its specific functions.

Sources

Foods that come from animals have a higher protein content than plant-derived sources. Meats contain approximately 80% of their energy from protein. It has been estimated that 65% of Americans get most of their protein from animal sources. Protein quality and quantity are different. Protein quantity refers to the amount of nitrogen found in food. Protein quality refers to the essential amino acid content in a protein compared with the needs of human cells. A protein that is able to provide all of the essential amino acids is known as a *complete protein*. Generally, this type of protein comes from an animal.

Animal Versus Plant Protein

Strong opinions often flare when comparing the quality of protein from animals vs that of plants, most vehemently from the vegetarian and vegan community. The development of the vegan and vegetarian movement is based primarily on passions without proper scientific findings, often citing cherry-picked data to back it up with what may seem like logic. The onus here is clearly on the vegan community to prove via randomized controlled studies that humans can increase muscles to their maximum potential in the same time frame as with animal-based proteins because that is essential for performance in athletes. The observational evidence is against this conjecture, as is research that shows animal sources are prevailing. The following are several facts concerning the comparison:

1. 30% of vegetarians are under-weight,[3] which is just as dangerous as being over-weight for mortality risk. This implies that even maintaining body weight is difficult with a vegetable-based diet.

2. Vegetarians (and especially vegans) are deficient in vitamin B_{12},[4-28] which is essential for nutrient utilization.

3. Vegetarian males by and large have depressed levels of 2 main hormones for muscle growth: testosterone[29-31] and IGF-1,[32-36] as well as having low levels of several amino acids necessary for tissue repair and growth.[37-47]

4. Vegetarians have a worse omega-6 to omega-3 profile than meat eaters.[48-52]

Of course, the issue is more complex than metabolic protein needs or meeting the recommended dietary allowance (RDA). Also note, articles of vegan nutrition conclude that amino acid quality and absorption is impaired in a vegan diet.[47] This makes trying to maintain health, never mind attempting to reach peak performance, difficult. These consistent findings would lead one to conclude that rare examples of vegan bodybuilders or competitive athletes in strength sports with any appreciable mass are extraordinary cases likely due to genetics, drug use, or false reporting of diet intake.

The origination of veganism or vegetarianism for overall health is debated. In fact, Corn Flakes were invented by John Harvey Kellogg to stop masturbation initially.[53] He felt that eating spicy, protein-rich foods lead to increased sexual arousal. He started the Sanitas Food Company to produce whole-grain cereals around 1897, a time when the standard breakfast for the wealthy was eggs and meat, while the poor ate porridge, farina, gruel, and other boiled grains because they were less expensive. Combined with influence from politicians and heavy media advertising, Kellogg published the 1927 *New Dietetics: A Guide to Scientific Feeding in Health and Disease*, which persuaded government officials to fundamentally change what was considered "healthy" breakfast from a primarily animal fat and protein breakfast to a vegan-friendly one, that being Kellogg's Corn Flakes. Not only did this false narrative prove to be the one Kellogg wanted to push on the public, it also meant a sharp rise in the increase of cereal profits as a "cheap and healthy" breakfast, as well as a correlative increase in cardiovascular disease.

There are multiple arguments to be made for consuming animal protein over plant protein for those with the proper genetic disposition for it. Foods that contain animal protein tend to be high in several nutrients that are often lacking in plant foods, such as the following:

* Vitamin B_{12}: A water-soluble vitamin that has a key role in the normal functioning of the brain and nervous system, and the formation of red blood cells.
* Docosahexaenoic acid (DHA): An essential omega-3 fat found in fatty fish such as salmon or mackerel. It is important for brain health and is hard to get from plant sources but can be found in flax, chia seeds, and seaweed.[54]
* Zinc: Found in animal protein sources such as beef, pork, and lamb. The largest benefit of eating animal protein-based foods containing zinc is that it is more easily absorbable.[55]
* Vitamin D: Vitamin D is found in oily fish, eggs, and dairy. Few plants contain it, but the type found in animal foods is better used by your body, similar to zinc.[56]

Essential nutrients like the ones previously mentioned show a marked difference in overall health between consuming animal protein and vegan-only sources of protein in an athlete's diet. For the layman or sedentary individual, lower levels of certain nutrients may not affect him or her negatively with symptoms for longer than athletes who are seeking peak performance. Therefore, it is recommended that athletes do not consume a vegan or vegetarian diet if their goal is to perform at the highest possible level for themselves individually.

How Much Protein Should an Athlete Consume?

There are vastly different opinions on how much protein we actually need. Most official nutrition organizations recommend a fairly modest protein intake. According to the US Dietary Guidelines, the RDA of 0.8 g of protein per kg of bodyweight. In the case of protein, the RDA of 0.8 g/kg is the minimum amount to avoid loss of lean muscle mass, which is the equivalent of about 56 g of protein for a sedentary average-sized adult male according to the Institute of Medicine; however, that was in 1960 when the average adult male was 154 lb. Today, according to the Centers for Disease Control and Prevention, the average adult male weights 195.5 lb[57] and, therefore, more general protein recommendations will have increased to 71 g.

In addition, that RDA is based on nitrogen balances and explained by the Institute of Medicine. Nitrogen balance is the difference between nitrogen intake and excreted nitrogen, measured by determining nitrogen lost in urine by a 24-hour urinary urea nitrogen test and comparing that to protein intake divided by 6.25. While this estimate may be accurate, it is also not particularly compelling. It is very easy to miscalculate adequate protein levels based on the nitrogen balance studies because they generally presume that your protein requirement is met when your nitrogen balance is zero. That particular assumption may lead to underestimating what a true protein requirement may be.

The United States Department of Agriculture (USDA) recommends about 2000 calories per day diet for average, moderately active women and about 2600 calories per day for moderately active men. The "reference" woman is 5'4" tall and weighs 126 lb and the "reference" man is 5'10" tall and weighs 154 lb. Again, these are not "average" weights for Americans before even considering body fat composition. The USDA also adheres to estimating that 10% to 35% of calories should come from protein. If a person on a 2000-calorie diet got 20% of calories from protein, that would equal 100 g/day. That number is almost twice as much as the typical American male that the US dietary guidelines recommend.

The reference woman would need 50 to 175 g of protein per day, and the reference man would need 65 to 228 g of protein per day. So, given this context, it is incredibly difficult to ascertain whether laypeople or athletes consume too much protein.

The US dietary guidelines may have actually made things more confusing because their protein recommendations are based on number of ounces. Granted, the recommendation is meant to cover everyone from young children to athletes to the elderly, but the problem is that the ounce equivalents really are not equal if you look up the grams of protein they have. A 1-oz chicken or steak equals about 8 to 9 g of protein, 1 oz of fish is about 6 g protein (and even this varies by the fish), and one egg has 6 g of protein. Once you go further and look at what is listed as "protein"-based foods that are not animals, the equivalency is worse. One tbsp of peanut butter has 4 g of protein and 1/4 cup of cooked beans has 4.2 g of protein. Therefore, if a woman following the above guidelines ate the recommended 5-oz equivalents of protein, she would get about 6 g/oz, for about 45 g/day.

There are also variations when getting into dairy-based sources of protein. One cup of 1% milk has 8 g of protein, 1 cup of low-fat yogurt has about 11 g, 1 cup of soy milk has 8 g, and 1.5 oz of natural cheese has 10 g, so when you add the dairy in, the average woman is getting about 27 more g of protein from the milk group, on top of the protein foods group.

The My Plate recommendations actually come out to be about 75 g of protein when you add dairy and other foods to the "protein foods" group for the "average" woman and 81 g of protein for "average" men. This is at the lower end of the guidelines of 10% to 35% of calories coming from protein. For a woman, 75 g of protein on a 2000-calorie diet is only 15% of calories from protein, and it is an even lower percentage, at 12% for a man on a 2600-calorie diet. These are the caloric recommendations in the US dietary guidelines for men and women with "moderate" activity levels, ages 26 to 45 years. The confusion reaches its peak when you realize that the guidelines estimate that we should monitor our sugar intake to be 10% or less of total calories, ultimately implying that sugar is about as important as protein in the diet.

Athletes' bodies need protein for many reasons, and if they do not get it through diet, their bodies will start breaking down muscle and other tissues in order to get protein. This leads to muscle wasting and weakness. Satisfactory protein is also required for bone health. You also need protein to form enzymes and to carry oxygen to tissues, so inadequate protein can cause lethargy. Low protein is also associated with hair loss, brittle nails, and cold hands and feet. A B_{12} deficiency (a vitamin only available in animal protein) has been shown as an independent risk factor for coronary artery disease and serious neurological disorders in infants of vegan mothers. Immune function decreases because protein is required for antibodies as stated previously.

TABLE 6-1		
DAILY PROTEIN FOODS		
	AGE	DAILY RECOMMENDATION
Children	2 to 3 years	2-oz equivalents
	4 to 8 years	4-oz equivalents
Girls	9 to 13 years	5-oz equivalents
	14 to 18 years	5-oz equivalents
Boys	9 to 13 years	5-oz equivalents
	14 to 18 years	6.5-oz equivalents
Women	19 to 30 years	5.5-oz equivalents
	31 to 50 years	5-oz equivalents
	51+ years	5-oz equivalents
Men	19 to 30 years	6.5-oz equivalents
	31 to 50 years	6-oz equivalents
	51+ years	5.5-oz equivalents

If we are being told to eat 0.8 g/kg of protein per kg of bodyweight, we are also being told by My Plate that nearly 60% of our dietary intake of protein should be in the form of dairy or soy milk products. It is extremely unclear how to determine how much protein to eat from meat, and the USDA recommendations do not really seem to be based on much science due to the inaccuracy of nitrogen balance studies and the gigantic ranges from the acceptable macronutrient distribution range, but a basic guideline shown here may help (Table 6-1).

It appears that 100 to 120 g of protein on a 2000-calorie diet is a very realistic amount for athletes to maintain muscle mass, assuming that does not put them into a large calorie deficit and they are not performing excessive exercise. Most athletes are eating much more than 2000/day, so of course they will need to increase that protein amount proportionately. To be clear, this recommendation of course is not a blanket statement, and individual requirements will vary greatly. The more salient point is if an athlete is having a protein-related problem such as low energy, inability to gain muscle, or increased adipose tissue, then their protein intake should be monitored for a reasonable length before making any specific or drastic changes to their diet. Appetite is a reliable driver to make sure you get enough protein to suit the athlete's needs. Appetite decreases when we get enough protein, so it is hard to eat too much protein because it is difficult to convert to energy. If athletes prioritize nutritious whole foods, changing protein intake is likely not going to be a diet modification that will allow athletes to create the body changes they seek.

CREATINE

by John Kiefer, MS

Creatine is the most significant sports supplement of the past 3 decades. This section examines a variety of benefits discovered through several well-controlled studies. However, most people—including supplement manufacturers and marketers—fail to understand what creatine does at the cellular level. In their material, as a result, they make false claims.

Creatine is powerful. Altering creatine levels affects your body at the most intimate and microscopic levels. This causes changes in nearly every cell in your body.

The real effects of creatine supplementation are demonstrated by it being the best-selling supplement ever. Creatine sales totaled over $100 million in 2016 alone, and these sales were to everyone from middle scholars to the elderly. With this recent rush of creatine madness, a wave of misinformation followed. The body of evidence concerning dosing, uses, and effect will be explained here not only so all the misinformation can be set straight, but also to elucidate what the actual science says.

What Is Creatine?

Creatine, physically, is a combination of 3 different amino acids: glycine, arginine, and methionine. As for what it does, I have read and heard countless times that creatine is the active transport of adenosine diphosphate (ADP) back into adenosine triphosphate (ATP). While vague, this concept is concise and impeachable. I have used this same explanation myself for the sake of avoiding further discussion simply because it is so elegant, but what does it mean?

First, a bit of history. Creatine is not a recent discovery. We have known about it for over 100 years,[58] and we have even known, for the majority of those 100 years, that supplementing with extra creatine can be beneficial.[59-61] Old-school supplementation entailed eating meat. In modern times, we can just buy a canister of grainy, white powder, mix it with water, and chug to our heart's content. Compared to what is possible naturally, this lets us take our creatine in mega-doses.

ATP is the energy currency of your cells, and ADP results from the breakdown of ATP, which releases a phosphate molecule and ADP. ADP is then recycled, a phosphate is reattached, and ATP is formed again. On the surface, it is a simple process.

Each of your cells contains mitochondria, which are dedicated energy producers. Mitochondria convert fatty acids, ketones, and glucose into ATP via the tricarboxylic acid (TCA) cycle, which you likely know as either the *Krebs cycle* or the *citric acid cycle*, depending on which textbook you are using and its country of origin.

At rest, mitochondria do not actually emit ATP or absorb ADP, which can be recycled into ATP in mitochondria.[62-65] Instead, creatine interacts with an enzyme system called **creatine kinase** (CK) that is located on the outer surface of mitochondria. It then picks up a phosphate molecule from ATP in the mitochondria, turning

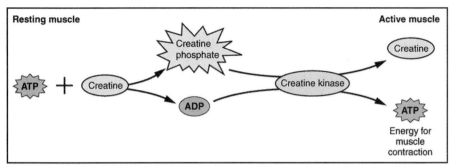

Figure 6-2. Interaction of mitochondria and CK. (Reprinted from https://commons.wikimedia.org/wiki/File%3A1016_Muscle_Metabolism.jpg. By OpenStax [CC BY 4.0 (http://creativecommons.org/licenses/by/4.0)], via Wikimedia Commons from Wikimedia Commons.)

the ATP into ADP.[66-70] Once the creatine grabs a phosphate, it is then called *creatine phosphate* (Figure 6-2).

Creatine phosphate then delivers the phosphate to the area of the cell that does work, where, once again, CK removes the phosphate from creatine phosphate and combines it with ADP at the source of work. This converts the ADP back into ATP. Essentially, creatine transports the energy produced by mitochondria directly to the working parts without invoking a long series of chemical steps. It is elegant, amazing, and efficient.

At its most basic level, creatine is the material that keeps all of our cells supplied with energy through a very efficient mechanism, while keeping intracellular ADP levels extremely low.

Quick Energy

It is important to keep intracellular ADP levels low because, as this concentration increases, cellular respiration decreases and can trigger the need for faster energy.[71-74] In other words, ADP buildup influences how soon the glycolytic cycle is turned on during intense bursts of work. By keeping ADP levels low and recycling ADP back into ATP at the site of work, you can produce peak power for a slightly longer period of time. This is the second major advantage of creatine within the cell.

When you try to produce a large amount of power in a very short time frame—during an Olympic lift, high-intensity repetitions, or the acceleration portion of a sprint—your muscle cells (especially your myofibrils) need excess energy fast. This is where the first of 3 energy systems come into play.

Cells have 3 energy systems. One of these is aerobic and the other 2 are anaerobic. Of the 2 anaerobic energy systems, most people know about the glycolytic system, where glucose is burned rapidly to produce ATP. The other, which actually kicks in before the glycolytic cycle, is the ATP-creatine-phosphate (ATP-CP) system.[75-78] When you ramp up power production quickly, your cells need ATP at a rate higher than free creatine can supply by grabbing a phosphate molecule and delivering it to the myofibril to get turned into ATP and then burned.

In contrast, when intense activity begins from rest, we already have a huge store of ATP and creatine phosphate. The cells burn through the ATP stores, and creatine phosphate recycles the resulting ADP into ATP rapidly, but CP becomes exhausted in the process. Within cells, ATP levels never fully deplete, even at fatigue. Creatine phosphate levels, however, can become almost totally exhausted.[79,80]

A Bigger Battery

Think of the ATP-CP system as a battery. During rest, your cells build a surplus of CP and ATP as it reaches equilibrium. Then, when it is go time, you can tap into this surplus for rapid, almost free energy because burning up the CP continues to prevent the buildup of ADP, which can decrease energy production when levels get too high.

This is one of the reasons why creatine supplementation gives you a boost. Supplementing with creatine can increase CP levels by roughly 20%.[81-83] This gives you a bigger battery when you need to produce massive amounts of power in very short periods of time.

This, however, is only a minor component. This battery is fast-acting, only lasting long enough for the glycolytic cycle to ramp up, which, in turn, only lasts long enough for the oxidative system to ramp up.[84,85] These 3 are not completely isolated—they all can contribute energy throughout exercise or work—but they each have a sweet spot where they produce the majority of the energy for the entire system.

Since ATP-CP acts on such a relatively short time frame (5 seconds[86]), it is critical for resistance-type training, sprinting, and high-intensity interval training. This can be seen through research: creatine supplementation does almost nothing to enhance endurance in performance,[87-91] but even relatively short exposure to supplementation can increase sprint and power performance.[92-100]

This is one of the instances when I will say that it is possible that supplementation beats training. Through various regulatory mechanisms—and from vast amounts of data on athletes, coupled with mathematical models—it does not seem possible to train the ATP-CP system directly. It is always tied with the peak output and timing of the glycolytic cycle.[101-103] Whatever the peak output is at which you train your lactic acid threshold, the ATP-CP system simply adjusts to reach the same exact peak, only in a shorter amount of time. In other words, the ATP-CP system only acts to bridge the first 5 seconds of high-output performance, in order to allow your glycolytic energy system to ramp up. Training may not be able to do anything to specifically alter the ATP-CP system in isolation. Supplementation, however, seems to have the ability to do this.

Muscular Hypertrophy

Creatine did not make such a massive splash in the supplement industry because of its ability to bridge energy systems and possibly help with getting 1 or 2 repetitions more than normal. Creatine supplementation is touted as an extremely effective muscle builder, and research supports this wholeheartedly,[104-113] which has been verified through meta-analysis.[114]

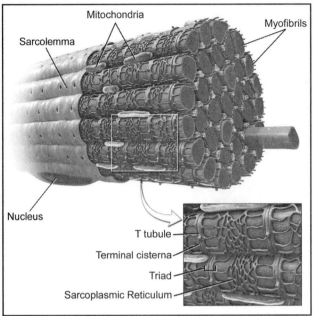

Mitochondria

Myofibrils

Sarcolemma

Nucleus

T tubule

Terminal cisterna

Triad

Sarcoplasmic Reticulum

Figure 6-3. Mitochondria within a myofibril. (Reprinted from Blausen.com staff (2014). "Medical gallery of Blausen Medical 2014". WikiJournal of Medicine 1 (2). DOI:10.15347/wjm/2014.010. ISSN 2002-4436. (Own work) [CC BY 3.0 (http://creativecommons.org/licenses/by/3.0)], via Wikimedia Commons from Wikimedia Commons.)

The myth spread by people who think any mass-market supplement must be junk—like your doctor—is that creatine supplementation does not increase lean body mass, but only increases fluid retention. If you are lucky, your neighborhood avid gym-goer who passes off word of mouth knowledge as fact will tell you the same thing. This is false. Creatine supplementation has been shown to cause a net flow of extra fluid into cells and even into the space between cells.[108,115] These intra- and extra-cellular pools do increase in fluid content,[116-118] but creatine does, in fact, increase muscle mass.

What is more curious is that even in the absence of resistance training, creatine supplementation can increase lean body mass.[113]

Creatine Is Anabolic

Remember, your body is in a constant state of protein turnover. It is constantly tearing down muscle tissue, then rebuilding it. The normal turnover rate for a lean, healthy individual is roughly 0.36 g of protein per pound of body weight (0.8 g/kg).[119,120] This means that a lean 200-lb male would need to consume at least 72 g of protein per day simply to maintain body mass. We shift this balance—even in the absence of resistance training—so the protein turnover is less and more protein is synthesized than destroyed, it would be possible to gain muscle taking in a small amount of protein. This is typically how anti-catabolic agents work. They do not increase growth signals per se, but they slow muscle protein breakdown. This is likely how creatine works to increase muscle size (Figure 6-3).

Creatine shifts the body's metabolism to grow more muscle by both increasing muscle protein synthesis and decreasing muscle protein breakdown. Specifically, creatine enhances growth of myosin heavy chain (MHC) type I and particularly type II fibers.[121-123] MHC type II fibers are the "fast twitch" muscle most responsible for the extreme amounts of muscle mass that one can achieve through resistance training.[124,125] This is particularly true for MHC IIa and IIx fibers.[126]

Note: You may have expected to read about MHC type IIb fibers like everyone else, including medical texts, but humans do not actually express the super-fast twitch fibers, type IIb. We possess a slightly slower counterpart called **type IIx**.[127]

Creatine Is Anti-Catabolic

Like I said, we can increase hypertrophy of muscle tissue in one of two ways: by increasing muscle protein synthesis (the anabolic process) and by decreasing muscle protein breakdown (the catabolic process). As I described, creatine is definitely anabolic by shifting toward greater protein synthesis. Creatine also slows muscle protein breakdown.

Creatine has been shown to decrease myostatin, one of the most catabolic and size-limiting genes in the human body.[128] By decreasing activation, you get a bump in the maximum size you can obtain. Theoretically, though, it should reach maximum effectiveness quickly. This coincides with the current rate of research, and it explains why creatine supplementation can be used to prevent muscle-wasting during old age and cancer treatment.[129,130]

Research has shown that creatine supplementation can increase muscle GLUT4 expression for up to 24 hours after resistance training above normal.[123,131-133] In short, the more GLUT4 transporters a muscle has, the greater its ability to absorb glucose, replenish glycogen stores, and prevent fat cells from storing glucose as part of body fat.

Researchers have also demonstrated that creatine supplementation can allow for supercompensation of glycogen levels within muscles, but only with resistance training.

Additionally, ingesting carbs can increase the retention of creatine levels within muscles.[134-136] If you eat a large bolus of carbs—especially fast-digesting carbs—the creatine boosts the response to carbs (in terms of glycogen storage) and the carbs boost the creatine retention.

After supplementing for a couple of weeks with creatine, the body burns more glucose than normal while at rest.[102] It is hard to say how this research translates from the case studied (the participants all ate a standard mixed diet), but if it does hold true, then through the non-carb portions of the day, the body may clear out glucose reserves faster.

Brain Boost and Longevity

Every cell in your body has mitochondria along with a creatine/creatine phosphate transport system, including the cells of the nervous system. By allowing an efficient and low-cost recycling system for ATP, creatine keeps cells running smoothly and allows them to navigate short-lived energy demands as though nothing has happened. This is true even in brain cells.[137,138] In a study that tested creatine supplementation in vegetarians, cognitive function was found to increase.[139,140] This is not surprising because vegetarians and vegans do not eat the primary dietary source of creatine (meat) and have lower levels than omnivores.[141] This is also likely why you never see vegans competing at a world-class level in power sports like sprinting or powerlifting. Creatine also helps fight against cognitive decline with age.[142]

There is evidence in rat models that suggests that creatine could increase lifespan.[143,144] Since we now know what creatine actually does in cells, this is not a surprising discovery. If your mitochondria do not need to do the extra work of converting ADP directly into ATP, we actually get a lower production of metabolic waste products. I am referring specifically here to positive ion carriers, which can put stress on the cellular machinery. The buildup of positive ion carriers is what causes fatigue in muscles, not excess lactate. Free potassium ($K+$), magnesium ($Mg+2$), and calcium ($Ca+2$), along with free hydrogen ($H+$, what lowers pH and increases acidity), are the sources of muscular fatigue.[145-148]

By supplementing with creatine, we prevent this excess mitochondrial respiration from activating, except during periods of physical exertion. During these periods, these effects can be beneficial, as you can see when you open any physique-oriented magazine and look at what results.

Supplementation Dosage

With scientific inquiry, sometimes the path we are on gets so worn down by the millions who came before us that it is easy to simply stay the course and do the same things we have always done. This is precisely what has happened regarding the use of creatine. Researchers kept using the same protocol for creatine supplementation after the first reports of successfully augmenting intramuscular creatine levels, and they are still using them today.

These studies found that 20 g/day of creatine, taken for 5 days, successfully raised muscle creatine content by 30% to 45%. The problem with the vast majority of these studies, however, is that they only lasted 5 to 7 days, yet we have been using them to make recommendations for people who supplement for months on end.

Note: I was not exhaustive in my search, but I pulled a large sample of research across different modes of inquiry (eg, looking for improvements in endurance, strength, power, and one-repetition max).

Of the 47 studies, only 4 tested or employed a protocol lasting longer than 14 days and attempted to use a maintenance dosage of creatine.[58-104] The idea in these studies is to load for 5 days at a high level—the standard 20 g/day—then maintain that supra-physiological concentration with 2 to 3 g daily thereafter. This protocol was first tested in 1996 with apparent positive results.[105] It has been used ever since.

This maintenance protocol should have seemed a bit suspect to other researchers, but only if they had taken the time to consider that a 150-lb male (approximately 70 kg) will burn through about 2 g of creatine naturally every day.[106] Since 95% of creatine exists within muscle tissue, the average resistance-trained athlete would require greater amounts of creatine just to maintain normal cellular levels.

It was not until 2003 that researchers tested this maintenance protocol using more advanced methods of determining intracellular creatine levels. The group found that after 2 weeks of using the standard maintenance protocol outlined previously, intracellular creatine levels returned to baseline.[104] In other words, the maintenance procedure did not maintain anything.

Note: The 2 g/day maintenance level is the current recommendation by the American College of Sports Medicine's expert panel on creatine.[107]

Unfortunately, there is no guiding research to be found regarding what it takes to actually maintain the supra-physiological values of intracellular creatine. All we know is that the current procedure is abysmal. I would guess, from examining the few dozen research papers available, that the amount you initially use is the daily dosage you should maintain.

As referenced earlier in the chapter, the majority of these papers simply used the standard 20 g/day mark without any rhyme or reason. This was an arbitrary choice by early investigators and, for some reason, it stuck. Only a handful of people used a formula that included bodyweight, but even they arrived at their conclusions by assuming that a 150-lb man should take 20 g of creatine per day. Again, nobody tested the assumption.

This cannot possibly be the optimal dosing schedule for everyone. On average, humans carry about 2 g of creatine per kg of lean muscle mass, which is about 1 g per pound. The maximum amount we can shove into muscles is about 3 g/kg (1.4 g/lb).[108] To hit this level, a 150-lb male would need about 25 g of creatine supplementation.

Because of the gap in research, I have to make some assumptions, but I will make reasonable ones. When we use these numbers to look at whole-body creatine status, we see that, in order to increase the amount of creatine we carry to a level above the baseline (1 g/lb), we need at least 2 g/day for maintenance, plus 0.4 g for every lean pound of muscle. Using the example of a 200-lb male with 10% body fat, we can give a rough estimate of at least 60 lbs of skeletal muscle. This would yield a reasonable calculation of (0.4 g/lb × 60 lbs)/0.95 + 2 g ≈ 27.3 g.

My hypothesis is that this would be the minimum amount of creatine needed on a daily basis to maintain maximum intracellular levels (the division by 0.95 takes into account the amount of creatine absorbed by the rest of the tissue in the body). This is the minimum daily amount needed because the well-controlled research shows that using the standard 2 g/day dosing returns intramuscular levels of creatine back to normal within 6 weeks.

There may be a better way to estimate the minimum daily dose, but the data do not exist to make a better recommendation. There is no need for a loading period if you are going by these formulas. If you are fairly lean, this leads to a simple formula to calculate your daily creatine intake:

* In lbs: Bodyweight × 0.15 = g of creatine monohydrate (CM) to ingest
* In kg: Body mass × 0.3 = g of CM to ingest

Even though I started from the actual difference in what muscles can hold, you will notice that these calculations give numbers that approximate the 20-g studies since many of the participants were around the 150-lb threshold. Unfortunately, the researchers did not extend their research to include the rest of the world.

Note: These formulas appear to overestimate needs, but since 1 g of CM is only 88% creatine, the overage takes this into account.

Creatine Sources

Creatine supplements come in several varieties: creatine ethyl ester (CEE), Kre-Alkalyn (KA; EFX Sports), CM, and even anhydrous creatine, which has nothing attached.

I will not go over all of these in too much detail because you can create as many versions as you want just by making a creatine "salt." For example, creatine citrate is a salt of creatine. None of these versions—if they have even been tested at all—have ever been tested to the degree of CM.

Creatine Monohydrate

In contrast to the others, CM is incredibly well-studied—and nearly every study referenced herein utilized CM. It is one of the most stable forms of creatine in solution, it is not degraded during normal digestion, and 99% is either absorbed by muscle tissue or excreted through sweat or urine.[109,110] It works, and it is cheap, too.

A few times now, I have mentioned the degradation of creatine in water. Creatine, when put into solution, will curl up into itself and create an inactive molecule called *creatinine*, which is a metabolic waste product. The first time I asked a doctor about creatine, he told me it was a waste product of metabolism, and that ingesting large doses of it would kill me. He was confusing creatine with creatinine, and his basic knowledge of cellular metabolism was, in fact, dangerously poor.

Creatine Ethyl Ester

This leads to our next version of creatine, CEE. Advertising hype behind CEE calls out to us from just about every magazine and website in existence, but that is all it is—hype. CEE degrades rapidly into creatinine in solution, and under normal physiological conditions (ingestion), most of it is converted rapidly and exclusively to creatinine.[111] Researchers even found a case where the rate of conversion of CEE to creatinine was so rapid that it caused false positives for liver disease.[112]

CEE is not an optimal vehicle to ingest creatine, and the only thing you should do with it is flush it down the toilet because you might actually poison yourself by taking it. At least my doctor may have been right about one form of creatine.

Salts

Through the citation of mysterious Bulgarian studies, the idea of a "buffered creatine" recently came into vogue, giving us the supplement known as KA. KA is actually a mixture of creatine salts, ash, and baking soda. You could recreate this stuff in your kitchen sink. Its manufacturer claims that KA produces a buffered solution of creatine that lasts longer before degrading, so more is ingested, making it 10 times more effective than CM. They claim, in fact, that 1.5 g of KA is equivalent to 10 to 15 g of CM.

Think about this. Your body, on a normal day, burns a minimum of 2 g of creatine. The makers of KA want you to believe that, although you are ingesting less than the minimum amount utilized by your body each day, it somehow magically morphs into the 20 to 30 g necessary to reach supra-physiological levels of intracellular creatine. They are counting on public ignorance for their marketing—a familiar tactic in the supplement industry, to be sure.

What about the idea of a buffered solution? By "buffered," the manufacturers mean one that will neutralize acidity, which will slow the degradation of creatine into creatinine. They claim that this buffering effect helps more creatine to pass through your stomach for utilization. What they fail to tell you, however, are 2 things:

1. CM, in water, creates an almost perfectly neutral solution, so no buffering is needed there before you ingest it.[113]

2. High acidity—such as the type in your stomach—actually blocks the conversion of creatine into creatinine, meaning once you swallow your CM, very little degrades into creatinine no matter how long it takes you to digest it.[109,114]

Now that we know something about the basic acid-base chemistry of creatine—and that none of the claims about KA could possibly be true or meaningful—we can look in one last place to see whether KA holds up: the peer-reviewed research. The Bulgarian studies are invalidated since nobody reviewed the research before it was published. The research that is actually peer-reviewed backs up the facts about KA that we already derived from a quick analysis of the basic chemistry of creatine: KA does not even remotely meet label claims and does not perform nearly as well as plain CM.[115]

Dosing Schedule

Daily dosage of creatine, as is the case in the majority of the research papers on the subject, is broken into 3 or 4 equal doses, taken every day throughout the day. Again, this protocol has never been directly tested to see if it is necessary to maintain supra-physiological levels of creatine.

One group of researchers did something interesting that suggests you do not need to take creatine all day long and that you do not need to take it every day as long as you are averaging the necessary amount per day.[116] Instead of taking 30 g/day, it may be possible to take 60 g every other day, achieving the same results. If anything, this research leads me to believe that taking creatine in divided doses all day long is probably unnecessary. If this is the case, we can better time when we ingest our creatine for maximal results.

How should this timing go? In general, you will want to time it around how you eat. Ingesting creatine with large amounts of carbs can actually increase retention of creatine within muscles.[117-120] Researchers have not explored the reasons for this, but they assume it has something to do with an interaction with insulin.[120]

Although I think they are on the right track, I think it actually has more to do with an interaction with GLUT4, which I will explain in a moment. For now, this tells us that, with carb back-loading in particular, the absolute best time to ingest creatine is immediately post-training with carbs. You could divide your daily dose amongst these meals, and if you are using CM, it is possible that one large load will do the job.

Avoid taking your creatine in the morning if you are a coffee drinker, or whenever you ingest caffeine. Creatine taken at the same time as caffeine, in the absence of carbs, can actually prevent a rise in intracellular creatine levels.[85,121] The common point of interaction, as surmised previously, may have something to do with the GLUT4 transporters since caffeine can prevent GLUT4 activation.

Creatine interacts with GLUT4 proteins in some way that has not been fully elucidated,[122,123] but what this does tell us is that anything that increases GLUT4 content and translocation (carbs and resistance training) will improve the results of supplementation, and anything that does not (caffeine and endurance training) will negate the effects. This also helps to explain why endurance athletes do not seem to receive any benefit whatsoever from creatine supplementation.

Do not take creatine with coffee. Do take creatine with training and/or carbs. Otherwise, take it however you would like.

Conclusion

Creatine is a powerful supplement, and it is not something that can easily be explained on the label of a bottle. For years now, we have been relying on supposition—and the arbitrary whims of the original researchers—to figure out how much to take and when to take it. This is poor science, and it is unfair to you, the practitioner and consumer who not only may be asked by athletes on how to use it, but may also be using it yourself. Now, you are armed with the knowledge to make intelligent choices regarding one of the few truly effective supplements on the market, free of poor science and supplement manufacturer propaganda.

CAFFEINE

Caffeine is a naturally occurring substance found in the beans, leaves, and fruit of various plants. It is most commonly ingested in the form of coffee, extracted from beans; tea, extracted from tea leaves; energy drinks from which the form typically is guarana seed or kola nut; and chocolate from cacao beans. It may also be bought in the anhydrous pill form and in mixed solutions of analgesics. It is the most commonly consumed drug in the world, and athletes frequently use it as an **ergogenic aid**. Figure 6-4 is a picture with common sources of caffeine and how much is in each one.

It improves endurance and performance during prolonged, moderately intense activity or exercise. To a lesser degree, it also enhances short-term, high-intensity athletic performance. Caffeine reduces the rate of perceived exertion,[149-153] improves concentration,[154,155] reduces fatigue, and enhances alertness. Routine caffeine consumption may cause tolerance or dependence, and abrupt discontinuation produces irritability, mood shifts, headache, drowsiness, or fatigue. Many major sport-governing bodies ban excessive use of caffeine; however, athletes may not even know it is possible to test positive for the supplement.

Note: Caffeine is a banned substance by the NCAA. A urinary caffeine concentration exceeding 15 mg/mL (corresponding to ingesting about 500 mg, the equivalent of 6 to 8 cups of brewed coffee, 2 to 3 hours before competition) results in a positive drug test.[156]

It is also important to understand that caffeine consumption can increase the effects of stimulant drugs such as amphetamines or methylphenidate (Ritalin, Concerta), causing nervousness, tremor, and insomnia. It can even counteract the anti-anxiety effects of medications like lorazepam. Practitioners should always be aware of what other medicine an athlete may be on if they are currently taking caffeine in any form.

Several mechanisms have been proposed to explain the physiologic effects of caffeine, but **adenosine receptor antagonism** most likely accounts for the primary mode of action. It is relatively safe according to the USDA and has no known negative performance effects, nor does it cause significant dehydration or electrolyte imbalance during exercise. An old study from 1928 began the notion that caffeine would cause dehydration, basing its conclusion on the fact that people who drank a lot of coffee tended to urinate more[157]; however, this was later shown to be caused by the absolute volume of fluid ingested and not caused by the actual caffeine.

Caffeine can increase the mobilization of fatty acids as a fuel during exercise.[158-167] It is the primary reason caffeine is popular among physique athletes.

Athletes do not typically take caffeine for the cholinomimetic properties that suppress appetite, the cognitive-enhancing abilities, the fat-burning properties, nor the claim it increases testosterone levels during training[168] or from raising your pain threshold. The most interesting effect of caffeine that athletes are likely not even aware of is the ability to decrease sensitivity to insulin.[169-177] Coupled with resistance training in the morning, caffeine (in the absence of a raise in insulin from carbs) will make fat and muscle cells resistant to insulin shuttling glucose into them, but muscle

Coffee	mg/cup	Drugs	mg/tab
Brewed ground	135	Actifed	0
Decaffeinated	5	Anacin	64
Drip	164	Aspirin (generic)	0
Instant	95	Bufferin	0
Percolated	134	Contac	0
		Dristan	30
Tea	**mg/5 oz**	Excedrin	130
Herbal	0	Midol	64
1-minute brew	21-33	NoDoz	200
3-minute brew	35-46	Triaminicin	30
5-minute brew	39-50	Tylenol	0
		Sudafed	0
Soft Drinks	**mg/12 oz**	Vanquish	66
Barqs Root Beer	22	Vivarin	200
Coke Classic	34.5		
Diet Coke	46.5	**Chocolate, cocoa, carob**	**mg/oz**
Dr. Pepper reg/diet	42	Baking chocolate	35
Fanta	0	Bittersweet chocolate	25
Fresca	0	Carob	0
Mountain Dew	55	Chocolate milk	6
Mr. Pibb	41	Cocoa mix drink	1
Mug Root Beer	0	Ovaltine	1
Pepsi Cola	37.5	Sweet/dark chocolate	20
Pepsi (sugar free)	36		
Sprite	0		
7-Up reg/diet	0		
Sunkist Orange	42		
Tab	45		

Figure 6-4. Average caffeine content of common foods, beverages, and medications.

cells are still able to intake glucose because the specific type of training translocates GLUT4 proteins to the surface of the cell, independent of insulin. This may be the most salient point regarding caffeine consumption and dovetails into how resistance training is effective to control or reverse type II diabetes. This modulated tissue response is a process by which we give each tissue of the body a specific instruction, either through diet, activity, or both.[178] Assumptions about one population cannot be applied to all populations out of context. Athletes (most of the time) are resistance-training heavy in one form or another. Someone who is overweight and inactive would be advised to stay away of the morning caffeine. For those athletes who do not resistance train, morning consumption of sugar and caffeine is accelerating insulin resistance and pancreatic overload. Once the GLUT4 translocate, they can transport sugar regardless of insulin levels. With caffeine and resistance training, you can control which tissues absorb glucose and which cannot at any time of day.[178]

Recommendations

* 3 to 5 mg of caffeine per kg of body weight will provide enhanced cognitive effects and energy without causing health risks. That means an average 70-kg athlete would only need 210 mg of caffeine, or a medium cup of regular coffee.

* More than 400 mg of caffeine at a time may cause irritability or other symptoms, so do not take too much at one time. Some studies have shown that up

to 1000 mg at a time may be safe,[179-184] but that is not recommended to test as individual tolerance will differ, as well as rate of metabolism.

* Caffeine can increase urinary calcium excretion. Consider limiting consumption or adding a calcium supplement, especially if an athlete has a bone injury.

* Effects of caffeine are noticeable 30 minutes after consumption, so time it properly to coincide with activity.

* Do not mix caffeine with other stimulants. This may cause a dangerous heart arrhythmia.

* Regular caffeine consumption will cause a tolerance build up, so chronic use for performance enhancement is not recommended.

* If cycling off caffeine, do not go cold turkey. If an athlete is used to drinking 2 cups of regular coffee per day, start with alternating between 2 cups and 1 cup per day for 5 to 7 days, then 1 cup/day, 1 cup every other day, etc. This will prevent symptoms of withdrawal such as headaches and daytime fatigue.

OTHER COMMON SUPPLEMENTS

Other than protein, creatine, and caffeine, there are several other common supplements that are used to a lesser extent by athletes to enhance performance. Supplement stores consistently bombard athletes with advertising and marketing campaigns in order to push their latest product. Since supplement companies are allowed to make any claims they want until proven otherwise, various outlandish advertisements hit the shelves at a dizzying speed.

Supplement claims are a double-edged sword. Some supplement companies will do one study on their product that shows drastic improvement for whatever it claims to do. Practitioners should always be questioning whether that study is legitimate, reproduceable, and applicable to an athlete's context of eating and activity. That one study may be compelling, but it is difficult to say it would be reproduceable without several similar studies coming to the same conclusion. That in and of itself would be difficult because supplement companies likely are not able to pay for multiple expensive studies to show that their product works, while still keeping the price of the product low enough to sell.

So many far-fetched claims have been made for supplements in recent years—especially the ones that help you drop body fat and/or build muscle—that people have come to believe that all supplements are just expensive placebos. Some supplements may be beneficial for those who otherwise do not get those particular nutrients or minerals in their daily diet. Some of the more common supplements are described in this chapter.

Essential Fatty Acids

Essential fatty acids (EFAs; ie, alpha-linoleic acid [omega-3] and linoleic acid [omega-6]) are both essential to the human diet. Those who limit fat intake for a host of reasons may not eat as many essential fats as they need for health and wellness. While alpha-linoleic acid (LNA) is listed as the essential form of the omega-3 fatty acids, the body has to convert it into DHA and eicosapentaenoic acid (EPA), the actual element of omega-3 fatty acids. Athletes can easily get enough of this in fatty fish, such as mackerel, sardines, and salmon. For those athletes who are allergic to fish or do not like to eat it, an EFA supplement may benefit them. If you do not get several servings of this type of fatty fish each week, you are probably deficient in omega-3 fats because your body cannot efficiently convert LNA into EPA and DHA.

Glucosamine and Chondroitin

Glucosamine and chondroitin have been widely promoted as a treatment for osteoarthritis. Chondroitin, a carb, is a cartilage component that is thought to promote water retention and elasticity and to inhibit the enzymes that break down cartilage. Supplements are generally made from cow cartilage. Glucosamine, an amino sugar, is supposed to promote the formation and repair of cartilage, and supplements are derived from shellfish shells. Both substances are created by the body.

They soothe the pain linked to sore joints and connective tissue and promote healing at a slow pace. The latter effect distinguishes the glucosamine-and-chondroitin combo from anti-inflammatory drugs, which relieve pain but do nothing to help repair tissue. That means it takes time for supplements aimed at joint treatment to work, based on cellular turnover speed. The typical doses are 1200 mg daily of glucosamine and 800 of chondroitin, which can be doubled initially.

The most well-known clinical trial came from the National Institute of Health, called the Glucosamine/chondroitin Arthritis Intervention Trial. In 2006, the researchers reported on a 24-week study that involved 1583 patients who were randomly assigned to receive 500 mg of glucosamine hydrochloride 3 times daily, 400 mg of sodium chondroitin sulfate 3 times daily, 500 mg of glucosamine plus 400 mg of chondroitin sulfate 3 times daily, 200 mg of celecoxib (Celebrex) daily, or a placebo. The study found that glucosamine and chondroitin, alone or together, did not reduce osteoarthritis knee pain more effectively than a placebo. The drug group did about 17% better than the placebo group.[185]

Chondroitin appears to be a placebo at best, and glucosamine has conflicting evidence, but the best-designed studies do not show a benefit.[186-189] To make matters more difficult, most product quality, quantity, and concentration are largely unknown.

Branched-Chain Amino Acids

Branched-chain amino acids (BCAAs) are made up of 3 essential amino acids: leucine, isoleucine, and valine. They are essential because the body is unable to make them out of other amino acids, meaning they must be ingested through food or supplements. These 3 amino acids make up about 40% of the daily requirement of all 9 essential amino acids, underscoring their importance. They are found in foods containing protein, with the highest concentrations in chicken, beef, eggs, salmon, and whey protein. They can also be supplemented, which can be useful for athletes because free-form BCAAs bypass the liver and gut tissue and go directly to the blood stream.

BCAAs have a branched side chain that initiates the job of converting each amino acid into energy during intense exertion. They make up about 35% of all muscle tissue. The more BCAAs that are present in the muscles, the more they will be used for energy, slowing the breakdown of muscles cells and preventing muscle loss.

How training and nutrition triggers muscle growth is an interesting process with many different components. The **mTOR** is one pathway that can signal the breakdown or growth of muscle tissue.[190] The mTOR target is a link in the chain that allows dietary components to activate the pathway of cellular hypertrophy. This is the interesting quality of the mTOR receptor. It ties dietary nutrients directly to the cellular signaling process.[191,192] Normally, hormones need to mediate these signals. For example, carbs cause a rise in insulin levels and insulin then potentiates the growth pathway (it will not cause growth without the necessary raw materials). Certain dietary supplements, however, can bypass the hormones and activate the pathway directly via mTOR. Just eating the right food triggers muscular hypertrophy. Leucine specifically binds to the mTOR receptor directly to trigger muscle growth and limit muscle breakdown.[193-195] That is why, of the 3 BCAAs, leucine is the one supplement that can be purchased as a stand-alone item.

Based on the pathways and mechanisms potentiated by leucine alone, it would be beneficial to time leucine supplementation to coincide with when nutrient uptake into muscles, such as after resistance training, for example. About 5 g of leucine will cause a very quick and high surge of insulin, helping to shuttle nutrients into muscle and triggering both anabolism and anti-catabolism.

Conclusion

Athletes take many supplements, as evidenced by the enormity of profits that supplement companies enjoy, whether they are beneficial or not. Several other common supplements could have been included here; however, these seem to be the most commonly used and researched. Although practitioners should always be pushing food over pill when an athlete is seeking a change, some supplements can be an effective alternative or catalyst when deemed appropriate.

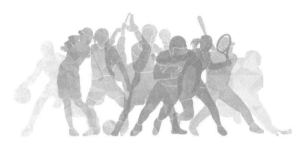

DEFINITIONS

Mammalian target of rapamycin (mTOR) pathway: An intracellular signaling pathway important in regulating the cell cycle; mTOR links with other proteins and serves as a core component of 2 distinct protein complexes, mTOR complex 1 and mTOR complex 2, which regulate different cellular processes including cell growth, proliferation, and motility

Creatine kinase: An enzyme, a protein necessary for muscle cells of the body to achieve their different chemical reactions

Type IIx: These fibers produce the most force but are incredibly inefficient based on their high myosin ATPase activity, low oxidative capacity, and heavy reliance on anaerobic metabolism

Ergogenic aid: Anything that gives you a mental or physical edge while exercising or competing

Adenosine receptor antagonist: A drug that acts as an antagonist of one or more of the adenosine receptors

mTOR: A protein kinase that links with other proteins and serves as a core component of 2 distinct protein complexes (mTOR complex 1 and mTOR complex 2), which regulate different cellular processes; in particular, as a core component of both complexes, mTOR functions as a serine/threonine protein kinase that regulates cell growth, cell proliferation, cell motility, cell survival, protein synthesis, autophagy, and transcription

REFERENCES

1. Six versions of Bill Number S.784 for the 103rd Congress. THOMAS.gov.
2. Dietary Supplements. FDA Office of Dietary Supplement Programs. Retrieved 1 July 2017.
3. Thorogood M, Appleby PN, Key TJ, et al. Relation between body mass index and mortality in an unusually slim cohort. *J Epidemiol Community Health.* 2003;57(2):130-133.
4. Mezzano D, Kosiel K, Martinez C, et al. Cardiovascular risk factors in vegetarians. Normalization of hyperhomocysteinemia with vitamin B(12) and reduction of platelet aggregation with n-3 fatty acids. *Thromb Res.* 2000;100(3):153-160.

5. Harman SK, Parnell WR. The nutritional health of New Zealand vegetarian and non-vegetarian Seventh-day Adventists: selected vitamin, mineral and lipid levels. *N Z Med J*. 1998;111(1062):91-94.
6. Donovan UM, Gibson RS. Dietary intakes of adolescent females consuming vegetarian, semi-vegetarian, and omnivorous diets. *J Adolesc Health*. 1996;18(4):292-300.
7. Janelle KC, Barr SI. Nutrient intakes and eating behavior scores of vegetarian and nonvegetarian women. *J Am Diet Assoc*. 1995;95(2):180-186, 189, quiz 187-188.
8. Larsson CL, Johansson GK. Dietary intake and nutritional status of young vegans and omnivores in Sweden. *Am J Clin Nutr*. 2002;76(1):100-106.
9. Krajcovicova-Kudlackova M, Blazicek P, Kopcova J, Bederova A, Babinska K. Homocysteine levels in vegetarians versus omnivores. *Ann Nutr Metab*. 2000;44(3):135-138.
10. Alexander D, Ball MJ, Mann J. Nutrient intake and haematological status of vegetarians and age-sex matched omnivores. *Eur J Clin Nutr*. 1994;48:538-546.
11. Bissoli L, Di Francesco V, Ballarin A, et al. Effect of vegetarian diet on homocysteine levels. *Ann Nutr Metab*. 2002;46(2):73-79.
12. Rauma AL, Torronen R, Hanninen O, Mykkanen H. Vitamin B-12 status of long-term adherents of a strict uncooked vegan diet ("living food diet") is compromised. *J Nutr*. 1995;125(10):2511-2515.
13. Lightowler HJ, Davies GJ. Micronutrient intakes in a group of UK vegans and the contribution of self-selected dietary supplements. *J R Soc Health*. 2000;120(2):117-124.
14. Lithell H, Vessby B, Hellsing K, et al. Changes in metabolism during a fasting period and a subsequent vegetarian diet with particular reference to glucose metabolism. *Ups J Med Sci*. 1983;88(2):109-119.
15. Sanders TA. Growth and development of British vegan children. *Am J Clin Nutr*. 1988;48(3 Suppl):822-825.
16. Sanders TA, Purves R. An anthropometric and dietary assessment of the nutritional status of vegan preschool children. *J Hum Nutr*. 1981;35(5):349-357.
17. Hellebostad M, Markestad T, Seeger Halvorsen K. Vitamin D deficiency rickets and vitamin B12 deficiency in vegetarian children. *Acta Paediatr Scand*. 1985;74(2):191-195.
18. Ashkenazi S, Weitz R, Varsano I, Mimouni M. Vitamin B12 deficiency due to a strictly vegetarian diet in adolescence. *Clin Pediatr (Phila)*. 1987;26(12):662-663.
19. Iamaroon A, Linpisarn S, Kuansuwan C. Iron and vitamin B12 deficiency anaemia in a vegetarian: a diagnostic approach by enzyme-linked immunosorbent assay and radioimmunoassay. *Dent Update*. 2002;29(5):223-224.
20. O'Gorman P, Holmes D, Ramanan AV, Bose-Haider B, Lewis MJ, Will A. Dietary vitamin B12 deficiency in an adolescent white boy. *J Clin Pathol*. 2002;55(6):475-456.
21. von Schenck U, Bender-Gotze C, Koletzko B. Persistence of neurological damage induced by dietary vitamin B-12 deficiency in infancy. *Arch Dis Child*. 1997;77(2):137-139. Review.
22. Herrmann W, Geisel J. Vegetarian lifestyle and monitoring of vitamin B-12 status. *Clin Chim Acta*. 2002;326(1-2):47-59. Review.
23. Hokin BD, Butler T. Cyanocobalamin (vitamin B-12) status in Seventh-day Adventist ministers in Australia. *Am J Clin Nutr*. 1999;70(3 Suppl):576S-578S.
24. Mann NJ, Li D, Sinclair AJ, et al. The effect of diet on plasma homocysteine concentrations in healthy male subjects. *Eur J Clin Nutr*. 1999;53(11):895-899.
25. Waldmann A, Koschizke JW, Leitzmann C, Hahn A. Homocysteine and cobalamin status in German vegans. *Public Health Nutr*. 2004;7(3):467-472.

26. Herrmann W, Schorr H, Obeid R, Geisel J. Vitamin B-12 status, particularly holo-transcobalamin II and methylmalonic acid concentrations, and hyperhomocystein-emia in vegetarians. *Am J Clin Nutr.* 2003;78(1):131-136.

27. Herrmann W, Schorr H, Purschwitz K, Rassoul F, Richter V. Total homocys-teine, vitamin B(12), and total antioxidant status in vegetarians. *Clin Chem.* 2001;47(6):1094-1101.

28. Sanders TA, Ellis FR, Dickerson JW. Haematological studies on vegans. *Br J Nutr.* 1978;40(1):9-15.

29. Habito RC, Ball MJ. Postprandial changes in sex hormones after meals of different composition. *Metabolism.* 2001;50(5):505-511.

30. Key TJ, Roe L, Thorogood M, Moore JW, Clark GM, Wang DY. Testosterone, sex hormone-binding globulin, calculated free testosterone, and oestradiol in male veg-ans and omnivores. *Br J Nutr.* 1990;64(1):111-119.

31. Howie BJ, Shultz TD. Dietary and hormonal interrelationships among vegetarian Seventh-Day Adventists and nonvegetarian men. *Am J Clin Nutr.* 1985;42(1):127-134.

32. Allen NE, Appleby PN, Davey GK, Kaaks R, Rinaldi S, Key TJ. The associations of diet with serum insulin-like growth factor I and its main binding proteins in 292 women meat-eaters, vegetarians, and vegans. *Cancer Epidemiol Biomarkers Prev.* 2002;11(11):1441-1448.

33. McCarty MF. Hepatic monitoring of essential amino acid availability may regulate IGF-I activity, thermogenesis, and fatty acid oxidation/synthesis. *Med Hypotheses.* 2001;56(2):220-224.

34. Takenaka A, Oki N, Takahashi SI, Noguchi T. Dietary restriction of single essential amino acids reduces plasma insulin-like growth factor-I (IGF-I) but does not affect plasma IGF-binding protein-1 in rats. *J Nutr.* 2000;130(12):2910-2914.

35. Noguchi T. Protein nutrition and insulin-like growth factor system. *Br J Nutr.* 2000;84(Suppl 2):S241-S244. Review.

36. McCarty MF. A low-fat, whole-food vegan diet, as well as other strategies that down-regulate IGF-I activity, may slow the human aging process. *Med Hypotheses.* 2003;60(6):784-792.

37. Steele M, Yokum D, Armstrong A. Efficacy of intraperitoneal amino acid (IPAA) dialysate in an Asian vegetarian patient with chronic hypoalbuminaemia. *EDTNA ERCA J.* 1998;24(2):28-32.

38. Shultz TD, Leklem JE. Nutrient intake and hormonal status of premenopausal veg-etarian Seventh-day Adventists and premenopausal nonvegetarians. *Nutr Cancer.* 1983;4(4):247-259.

39. Ball MJ, Bartlett MA. Dietary intake and iron status of Australian vegetarian women. *Am J Clin Nutr.* 1999;70(3):353-358.

40. Laidlaw SA, Shultz TD, Cecchino JT, Kopple JD. Plasma and urine taurine levels in vegans. *Am J Clin Nutr.* 1988;47(4):660-663.

41. Rana SK, Sanders TA. Taurine concentrations in the diet, plasma, urine and breast milk of vegans compared with omnivores. *Br J Nutr.* 1986;56(1):17-27.

42. Okuda T, Miyoshi-Nishimura H, Makita T, et al. Protein metabolism in vegans. *Ann Physiol Anthropol.* 1994;13(6):393-401.

43. Donaldson MS. Metabolic vitamin B12 status on a mostly raw vegan diet with follow-up using tablets, nutritional yeast, or probiotic supplements. *Ann Nutr Metab.* 2000;44(5-6):229-234.

44. Acosta PB. Availability of essential amino acids and nitrogen in vegan diets. *Am J Clin Nutr.* 1988;48(3 Suppl):868-874. Review.

45. Vargas E, Bressani R, Navarrete DA, Braham JE, Elias LG. A new alternative for estimating recommendations of protein intake in humans. Protein requirements of an adult population fed with a diet based on rice and beans. *Arch Latinoam Nutr.* 1985;35(3):394-405.

46. Massa G, Vanoppen A, Gillis P, Aerssens P, Alliet P, Raes M. Protein malnutrition due to replacement of milk by rice drink. *Eur J Pediatr.* 2001;160(6):382-384.

47. Caso G, Scalfi L, Marra M, et al. Albumin synthesis is diminished in men consuming a predominantly vegetarian diet. *J Nutr.* 2000;130(3):528-533.

48. Krajcovicova-Kudlackova M, Blazicek P, Babinska K, et al. Traditional and alternative nutrition--levels of homocysteine and lipid parameters in adults. *Scand J Clin Lab Invest.* 2000;60:657-664.

49. Strucinska M. Vegetarian diets of breastfeeding women in the light of dietary recommendations. *Rocz Panstw Zakl Hig.* 2002;53(1):65-79. Review.

50. Shultz TD, Leklem JE. Nutrient intake and hormonal status of premenopausal vegetarian Seventh-day Adventists and premenopausal nonvegetarians. *Nutr Cancer.* 1983;4(4):247-259.

51. Agren JJ, Tormala ML, Nenonen MT, Hanninen OO. Fatty acid composition of erythrocyte, platelet, and serum lipids in strict vegans. *Lipids.* 1995;30(4):365-369.

52. Roshanai F, Sanders TA. Assessment of fatty acid intakes in vegans and omnivores. *Hum Nutr Appl Nutr.* 1984;38(5):345-354.

53. Damour L, Hansell J. *Abnormal Psychology.* 2nd ed. NJ: John Wiley & Sons, Inc; 2008:368.

54. Gebauer S, Psota T, Harris W, et al. n-3 fatty acid dietary recommendations and food sources to achieve essentiality and cardiovascular benefits. *Am J Clin Nutr.* 2006;83(6 Suppl):1526S-1535S.

55. Cotton P, Subar A, Friday J, et al. Dietary sources of nutrients among US adults, 1994 to 1996. *J Am Diet Assoc.* 2004;104(6):921-930.

56. Romagnoli E, Mascia M, Cipriani C, et al. Short and long-term variations in serum calciotropic hormones after a single very large dose of ergocalciferol (vitamin D2) or cholecalciferol (vitamin D3) in the elderly. *J Clin Endocrinol Metab.* 2008;93(8):3015-3020. doi: 10.1210/jc.2008-0350.

57. Centers for Disease Control. Health, United States, 2016. Available from: https://www.cdc.gov/nchs/hus/contents2016.htm#053

58. Folin O, Denis W. Protein metabolism from the standpoint of blood tissue analysis: third paper; further absorption experiments with especial reference to the behavior of creatine and creatinine and to the formation of urea. *J Biol Chem.* 1912;12:141-162.

59. Bloch K, Shoenheimer R. The metabolic relation of creatine and creatinine studied with isotopic nitrogen. *J BioZ Chem.* 1939;131:111-118.

60. Chanutin A. The fate of creatine when administered to man. *J Biol Chem.* 1926;67:29-34.

61. Hoberman HD, Sims EA, Peters JH. Creatine and creatinine metabolism in the normal male adult studied with the aid of isotopic nitrogen. *J BioZ Chem.* 1948;172:45-51.

62. Klingenberg M, Pfaff E. In Tager JM, ed. *Regulation of Metabolic Processes in Mitochondria.* Amsterdam, the Netherlands: Elsevier; 1966:180.

63. Meisner H, Klingenberg M. Efflux of adenine nucleotides from rat liver mitochondria. *J Biol Chem.* 1968;243(13):3631-3639.

64. Klingenberg M. The ADP-ATP translocation in mitochondria, a membrane potential controlled transport. *J Membr Biol.* 1980;56(2):97-105. Review.

65. Klingenberg M. The ADP and ATP transport in mitochondria and its carrier. *Biochim Biophys Acta.* 2008;1778(10):1978-2021.

66. Bessman SP, Geiger PJ. Transport of energy in muscle: the phosphorylcreatine shuttle. *Science*. 1981;211(4481):448-452. Review.
67. Wallimann T. Bioenergetics. Dissecting the role of creatine kinase. *Curr Biol*. 1994;4(1):42-46.
68. Meyer RA, Sweeney HL, Kushmerick MJ. A simple analysis of the "phosphocreatine shuttle." *Am J Physiol Cell Physiol*. 1984;246:C365-C377.
69. Perry CG, Kane DA, Herbst EA, et al. Mitochondrial creatine kinase activity and phosphate shuttling are acutely regulated by exercise in human skeletal muscle. *J Physiol*. 2012;590(Pt 21):5475-5486.
70. Bessman SP. The creatine-creatine phosphate energy shuttle. *Annu Rev Biochem*. 1985;54:831-862.
71. Balaban RS. Regulation of oxidative phosphorylation in the mammalian cell. *Am J Physiol*. 1990;258(3 Pt 1):C377-C389. Review.
72. Korzeniewski B. Theoretical studies on the regulation of oxidative phosphorylation in intact tissues. *Biochim Biophys Acta*. 2001;1504(1):31-45. Review.
73. From AH, Zimmer SD, Michurski SP, et al. Regulation of the oxidative phosphorylation rate in the intact cell. *Biochemistry*. 1990;29(15):3731-3743.
74. Saks VA, Kongas O, Vendelin M, Kay L. Role of the creatine/phosphocreatine system in the regulation of mitochondrial respiration. *Acta Physiol Scand*. 2000;168(4):635-641.
75. Bangsbo J, Graham TE, Kiens B, Saltin B. Elevated muscle glycogen and anaerobic energy production during exhaustive exercise in man. *J Physiol*. 1992;451:205-227.
76. Smith JC, Hill DW. Contribution of energy systems during a Wingate power test. *Br J Sports Med*. 1991;25(4):196-199.
77. Serresse O, Simoneau JA, Bouchard C, Boulay MR. Aerobic and anaerobic energy contribution during maximal work output in 90 s determined with various ergocycle workloads. *Int J Sports Med*. 1991;12(6):543-547.
78. Boulay MR, Lortie G, Simoneau JA, Hamel P, Leblanc C, Bouchard C. Specificity of aerobic and anaerobic work capacities and powers. *Int J Sports Med*. 1985;6(6):325-328.
79. Bangsbo J, Madsen K, Kiens B, Richter EA. Effect of muscle acidity on muscle metabolism and fatigue during intense exercise in man. *J Physiol*. 1996;495(Pt 2):587-596.
80. Sargeant AJ. Structural and functional determinants of human muscle power. *Exp Physiol*. 2007;92(2):323-331. Epub 2007 Jan 25. Review.
81. Greenhaff PL, Bodin K, Soderlund K, Hultman E. Effect of oral creatine supplementation on skeletal muscle phosphocreatine resynthesis. *Am J Physiol*. 1994;266(5 Pt 1):E725-E730.
82. Harris RC, Söderlund K, Hultman E. Elevation of creatine in resting and exercised muscle of normal subjects by creatine supplementation. *Clin Sci (Lond)*. 1992;83(3):367-374.
83. Hultman E, Söderlund K, Timmons JA, Cederblad G, Greenhaff PL. Muscle creatine loading in men. *J Appl Physiol*. 1996;81(1):232-237.
84. Bangsbo J, Krustrup P, González-Alonso J, Saltin B. ATP production and efficiency of human skeletal muscle during intense exercise: effect of previous exercise. *Am J Physiol Endocrinol Metab*. 2001;280(6):E956-E964.
85. Smith JC, Hill DW. Contribution of energy systems during a Wingate power test. *Br J Sports Med*. 1991;25(4):196-199.
86. Maughan RJ, Gleeson M, Greenhaff PL. *Biochemistry of Exercise and Training*. Oxford: Oxford University Press; 1997.

87. Terjung RL, Clarkson P, Eichner ER, et al. American College of Sports Medicine roundtable. The physiological and health effects of oral creatine supplementation. *Med Sci Sports Exerc.* 2000;32(3):706-717.

88. Balsom PD, Harridge SD, Soderlund K, Sjodin B, Ekblom B. Creatine supplementation per se does not enhance endurance exercise performance. *Acta Physiol Scand.* 1993;149(4):521-523.

89. Engelhardt M, Neumann G, Berbalk A, Reuter I. Creatinine supplementation in endurance sports. *Med Sci Sports Exerc.* 1998;30:1123-1129.

90. Cooper R, Naclerio F, Allgrove J, Jimenez A. Creatine supplementation with specific view to exercise/sports performance: an update. *J Int Soc Sports Nutr.* 2012;9(1):33.

91. Vandebuerie F, Vanden Eynde B, Vandenberghe K, Hespel P. Effect of creatine loading on endurance capacity and sprint power in cyclists. *Int J Sports Med.* 1998;19(7):490-495.

92. Greenhaff PL, Casey A, Short AH, Harris R, Soderlund K, Hultman E. Influence of oral creatine supplementation of muscle torque during repeated bouts of maximal voluntary exercise in man. *Clin Sci (Lond).* 1993;84(5):565-571.

93. Kilduff LP, Vidakovic P, Cooney G, et al. Effects of creatine on isometric bench-press performance in resistance-trained humans. *Med Sci Sports Exerc.* 2002;34(7):1176-1183.

94. Becque MD, Lochmann JD, Melrose DR. Effects of oral creatine supplementation on muscular strength and body composition. *Med Sci Sports Exerc.* 2000;32(3):654-658.

95. Balsom, PD, Ekblom B, Soderlund K, Sjodin B, Hultman, E. Creatine supplementation and dynamic high-intensity exercise. *Scand J Med Sci Sports.* 1993;3:143-149.

96. Becque M, Lochmann JD, Melrose D. Effect of creatine supplementation during strength training on 1-RM and body composition. *Med Sci Sports Exerc.* 1997;29:S146.

97. Balsom PD, Soderlund K, Sjodin B, Ekblom B. Skeletal muscle metabolism during short duration high-intensity exercise: influence of creatine supplementation. *Acta Physiol Scand.* 1995;154(3):303-310.

98. Hoffman JR, Stout JR, Falvo MJ, Kang J, Ratamess NA. Effect of low-dose, short-duration creatine supplementation on anaerobic exercise performance. *J Strength Cond Res.* 2005;19(2):260-264.

99. Smith JC, Stephens DP, Hall EL, Jackson AW, Earnest CP. Effect of oral creatine ingestion on parameters of the work rate-time relationship and time to exhaustion in high-intensity cycling. *Eur J Appl Physiol Occup Physiol.* 1998;77(4):360-365.

100. Kreider RB, Ferreira M, Wilson M, et al. Effects of creatine supplementation on body composition, strength, and sprint performance. *Med Sci Sports Exerc.* 1998;30(1):73-82.

101. Gastin PB, Lawson DL. Influence of training status on maximal accumulated oxygen deficit during all-out exercise. *Eur J Appl Physiol.* 1994;69:321-330.

102. Baker JS, McCormick MC, Robergs RA. Interaction among skeletal muscle metabolic energy systems during intense exercise. *J Nutr Metab.* 2010;2010:905612.

103. Gastin PB. Energy system interaction and relative contribution during maximal exercise. *Sports Med.* 2001;31(10):725-741. Review.

104. Candow DG, Chilibeck PD, Chad KE, Chrusch MJ, Davison KS, Burke DG. Effect of ceasing creatine supplementation while maintaining resistance training in older men. *J Aging Phys Act.* 2004;12(3):219-231.

105. Saremi A, Gharakhanloo R, Sharghi S, Gharaati MR, Larijani B, Omidfar K. Effects of oral creatine and resistance training on serum myostatin and GASP-1. *Mol Cell Endocrinol.* 2010;317(1-2):25-30.

106. Volek JS, Ratamess NA, Rubin MR, et al. The effects of creatine supplementation on muscular performance and body composition responses to short-term resistance training overreaching. *Eur J Appl Physiol.* 2004;91(5-6):628-637.

107. Bemben MG, Lamont HS. Creatine supplementation and exercise performance: recent findings. *Sports Med.* 2005;35(2):107-125. Review.

108. Balsom PD, Söderlund K, Ekblom B. Creatine in humans with special reference to creatine supplementation. *Sports Med.* 1994;18(4):268-280. Review.

109. van Loon LJ, Oosterlaar AM, Hartgens F, Hesselink MK, Snow RJ, Wagenmakers AJ. Effects of creatine loading and prolonged creatine supplementation on body composition, fuel selection, sprint and endurance performance in humans. *Clin Sci (Lond).* 2003;104(2):153-162.

110. Cooke WH, Grandjean PW, Barnes WS. Effect of oral creatine supplementation on power output and fatigue during bicycle ergometry. *J Appl Physiol.* 1995;78(2):670-673.

111. Green AL, Hultman E, Macdonald IA, Sewell DA, Greenhaff PL. Carbohydrate ingestion augments skeletal muscle creatine accumulation during creatine supplementation in humans. *Am J Physiol.* 1996;271(5 Pt 1):E821-E826.

112. Mujika I, Chatard JC, Lacoste L, Barale F, Geyssant A. Creatine supplementation does not improve sprint performance in competitive swimmers. *Med Sci Sports Exerc.* 1996;28(11):1435-1441.

113. van Loon LJ, Oosterlaar AM, Hartgens F, Hesselink MK, Snow RJ, Wagenmakers AJ. Effects of creatine loading and prolonged creatine supplementation on body composition, fuel selection, sprint and endurance performance in humans. *Clin Sci (Lond).* 2003;104(2):153-162.

114. Branch JD. Effect of creatine supplementation on body composition and performance: a meta-analysis. *Int J Sport Nutr Exerc Metab.* 2003;13(2):198-226.

115. Juhn MS, Tarnopolsky M. Potential side effects of oral creatine supplementation: a critical review. *Clin J Sport Med.* 1998;8(4):298-304. Review.

116. Easton C, Turner S, Pitsiladis YP. Creatine and glycerol hyperhydration in trained subjects before exercise in the heat. *Int J Sport Nutr Exerc Metab.* 2007;17(1):70-91.

117. Weiss BA, Powers ME. Creatine supplementation does not impair the thermoregulatory response during a bout of exercise in the heat. *J Sports Med Phys Fitness.* 2006;46(4):555-563.

118. Kilduff LP, Georgiades E, James N, et al. The effects of creatine supplementation on cardiovascular, metabolic, and thermoregulatory responses during exercise in the heat in endurance-trained humans. *Int J Sport Nutr Exerc Metab.* 2004;14(4):443-460.

119. Rand WM, Pellett PL, Young VR. Meta-analysis of nitrogen balance studies for estimating protein requirements in healthy adults. *Am J Clin Nutr.* 2003;77(1):109-127.

120. Trumbo P, Schlicker S, Yates AA, Poos M; Food and Nutrition Board of the Institute of Medicine, The National Academies. Dietary reference intakes for energy, carbohydrate, fiber, fat, fatty acids, cholesterol, protein and amino acids. *J Am Diet Assoc.* 2002;102(11):1621-1630.

121. Willoughby DS, Rosene JM. Effects of oral creatine and resistance training on myogenic regulatory factor expression. *Med Sci Sports Exerc.* 2003;35(6):923-929.

122. Willoughby DS, Rosene J. Effects of oral creatine and resistance training on myosin heavy chain expression. *Med Sci Sports Exerc.* 2001;33(10):1674-1681.

123. Deldicque L, Atherton P, Patel R, et al. Effects of resistance exercise with and without creatine supplementation on gene expression and cell signaling in human skeletal muscle. *J Appl Physiol.* 2008;104(2):371-378.

124. Schiaffino S, Reggiani C. Fiber types in mammalian skeletal muscles. *Physiol Rev.* 2011;91(4):1447-531.

125. Harridge SD, Bottinelli R, Canepari M, et al. Whole-muscle and single-fibre contractile properties and myosin heavy chain isoforms in humans. *Pflugers Arch.* 1996;432(5):913-920.

126. D'Antona G, Lanfranconi F, Pellegrino MA, et al. Skeletal muscle hypertrophy and structure and function of skeletal muscle fibres in male body builders. *J Physiol.* 2006;570(Pt 3):611-627.

127. Pette D, Peuker H, Staron RS. The impact of biochemical methods for single muscle fibre analysis. *Acta Physiol Scand.* 1999;166(4):261-277. Review.

128. Saremi A, Gharakhanloo R, Sharghi S, Gharaati MR, Larijani B, Omidfar K. Effects of oral creatine and resistance training on serum myostatin and GASP-1. *Mol Cell Endocrinol.* 2010;317(1-2):25-30.

129. Tarnopolsky MA. Clinical use of creatine in neuromuscular and neurometabolic disorders. *Subcell Biochem.* 2007;46:183-204. Review.

130. Sakkas GK, Schambelan M, Mulligan K. Can the use of creatine supplementation attenuate muscle loss in cachexia and wasting? *Curr Opin Clin Nutr Metab Care.* 2009;12(6):623-627. Review.

131. van Loon LJ, Murphy R, Oosterlaar AM, et al. Creatine supplementation increases glycogen storage but not GLUT-4 expression in human skeletal muscle. *Clin Sci (Lond).* 2004;106(1):99-106.

132. Derave W, Eijnde BO, Verbessem P, et al. Combined creatine and protein supplementation in conjunction with resistance training promotes muscle GLUT-4 content and glucose tolerance in humans. *J Appl Physiol.* 2003;94(5):1910-1916.

133. Op 't Eijnde B, Ursø B, Richter EA, Greenhaff PL, Hespel P. Effect of oral creatine supplementation on human muscle GLUT4 protein content after immobilization. *Diabetes.* 2001;50(1):18-23.

134. Steenge GR, Simpson EJ, Greenhaff PL. Protein- and carbohydrate-induced augmentation of whole body creatine retention in humans. *J Appl Physiol.* 2000;89(3):1165-1171.

135. Green AL, Simpson EJ, Littlewood JJ, Macdonald IA, Greenhaff PL. Carbohydrate ingestion augments creatine retention during creatine feeding in humans. *Acta Physiol Scand.* 1996;158(2):195-202.

136. Pittas G, Hazell MD, Simpson EJ, Greenhaff PL. Optimization of insulin-mediated creatine retention during creatine feeding in humans. *J Sports Sci.* 2010;28(1):67-74.

137. Sappey-Marinier D, Calabrese G, Fein G, Hugg JW, Biggins C, Weiner MW. Effect of photic stimulation on human visual cortex lactate and phosphates using 1H and 31P magnetic resonance spectroscopy. *J Cereb Blood Flow Metab.* 1992;12(4):584-592.

138. Rango M, Castelli A, Scarlato G. Energetics of 3.5 s neural activation in humans: a 31P MR spectroscopy study. *Magn Reson Med.* 1997;38(6):878-883.

139. Rae C, Digney AL, McEwan SR, Bates TC. Oral creatine monohydrate supplementation improves brain performance: a double-blind, placebo-controlled, cross-over trial. *Proc Biol Sci.* 2003;270(1529):2147-2150.

140. Benton D, Donohoe R. The influence of creatine supplementation on the cognitive functioning of vegetarians and omnivores. *Br J Nutr.* 2011;105(7):1100-1105.

141. Delanghe J, De Slypere JP, De Buyzere M, Robbrecht J, Wieme R, Vermeulen A. Normal reference values for creatine, creatinine, and carnitine are lower in vegetarians. *Clin Chem.* 1989;35(8):1802-1803.

142. McMorris T, Mielcarz G, Harris RC, Swain JP, Howard A. Creatine supplementation and cognitive performance in elderly individuals. *Neuropsychol Dev Cogn B Aging Neuropsychol Cogn.* 2007;14(5):517-528.

143. Klopstock T, Elstner M, Bender A. Creatine in mouse models of neurodegeneration and aging. *Amino Acids.* 2011;40(5):1297-1303. Review.

144. Bender A, Beckers J, Schneider I, et al. Creatine improves health and survival of mice. *Neurobiol Aging.* 2008;29(9):1404-1411.

145. Halestrap AP, Griffiths EJ, Connern CP. Mitochondrial calcium handling and oxidative stress. *Biochem Soc Trans.* 1993;21(2):353-358. Review.

146. Bangsbo J, Juel C, Hellsten Y, Saltin B. Dissociation between lactate and proton exchange in muscle during intense exercise in man. *J Physiol.* 1997;504(Pt 2):489-499.

147. McKenna MJ, Heigenhauser GJ, McKelvie RS, MacDougall JD, Jones NL. Sprint training enhances ionic regulation during intense exercise in men. *J Physiol.* 1997;501(Pt 3):687-702.

148. Huso ME, Hampl JS, Johnston CS, Swan PD. Creatine supplementation influences substrate utilization at rest. *J Appl Physiol (1985).* 2002;(6):2018-2022.

149. Beaven CM, Hopkins WG, Hansen KT, Wood MR, Cronin JB, Lowe TE. Dose effect of caffeine on testosterone and cortisol responses to resistance exercise. *Int J Sport Nutr Exerc Metab.* 2008;18(2):131-141.

150. Umemura T, Ueda K, Nishioka K, et al. Effects of acute administration of caffeine on vascular function. *Am J Cardiol.* 2006;98(11):1538-1541.

151. Davis JK, Green JM. Caffeine and anaerobic performance: ergogenic value and mechanisms of action. *Sports Med.* 2009;39(10):813-832.

152. Tarnopolsky MA. Effect of caffeine on the neuromuscular system—potential as an ergogenic aid. *Appl Physiol Nutr Metab.* 2008;33(6):1284-1289.

153. Green JM, Wickwire PJ, McLester JR, et al. Effects of caffeine on repetitions to failure and ratings of perceived exertion during resistance training. *Int J Sports Physiol Perform.* 2007;2(3):250-259.

154. Tse SY. Coffee contains cholinomimetic compound distinct from caffeine. I: Purification and chromatographic analysis. *J Pharm Sci.* 1991;80(7):665-669.

155. Tse SY. Cholinomimetic compound distinct from caffeine contained in coffee. II: Muscarinic actions. *J Pharm Sci.* 1992;81(5):449-452.

156. The National Collegiate Athletic Association. 2017-2018 list of banned NCAA substances. NCAA.org. http://www.ncaa.org/2017-18-ncaa-banned-drugs-list. Accessed October 11, 2017.

157. Candilio L, Chen A, Iqbal R, et al. An interesting case of tachyarrhythmia. *BMJ Case Reports.* 2014; doi:10.1136/bcr-2014-205481.

158. Jung RT, Shetty PS, James WP, Barrand MA, Callingham BA. Caffeine: its effect on catecholamines and metabolism in lean and obese humans. *Clin Sci (Lond).* 1981;60(5):527-535.

159. Arciero PJ, Gardner AW, Calles-Escandon J, Benowitz NL, Poehlman ET. Effects of caffeine ingestion on NE kinetics, fat oxidation, and energy expenditure in younger and older men. *Am J Physiol.* 1995;268(6 Pt 1):E1192-E1198.

160. Ivy JL, Costill DL, Fink WJ, Lower RW. Influence of caffeine and carbohydrate feedings on endurance performance. *Med Sci Sports.* 1979;11(1):6-11.

161. Acheson KJ, Gremaud G, Meirim I, et al. Metabolic effects of caffeine in humans: lipid oxidation or futile cycling? *Am J Clin Nutr.* 2004;79(1):40-46.

162. Mougios V, Ring S, Petridou A, Nikolaidis MG. Duration of coffee- and exercise-induced changes in the fatty acid profile of human serum. *J Appl Physiol.* 2003;94(2):476-484.

163. Hetzler RK, Knowlton RG, Somani SM, Brown DD, Perkins RM 3rd. Effect of parax-anthine on FFA mobilization after intravenous caffeine administration in humans. *J Appl Physiol.* 1990;68(1):44-47.

164. Goldrick RB, McLoughlin GM. Lipolysis and lipogenesis from glucose in human fat cells of different sizes. Effects of insulin, epinephrine, and theophylline. *J Clin Invest.* 1970;49(6):1213-1223.

165. Raguso CA, Coggan AR, Sidossis LS, Gastaldelli A, Wolfe RR. Effect of theophylline on substrate metabolism during exercise. *Metabolism.* 1996;45(9):1153-1160.

166. Peters EJ, Klein S, Wolfe RR. Effect of short-term fasting on the lipolytic response to theophylline. *Am J Physiol.* 1991;261(4 Pt 1):E500-E504.

167. Acheson KJ, Zahorska-Markiewicz B, Pittet P, Anantharaman K, Jequier E. Caffeine and coffee: their influence on metabolic rate and substrate utilization in normal weight and obese individuals. *Am J Clin Nutr.* 1980;33(5):989-997.

168. REF 1 Beaven CM, Hopkins WG, Hansen KT, Wood MR, Cronin JB, Lowe TE. Dose effect of caffeine on testosterone and cortisol responses to resistance exercise. *Int J Sport Nutr Exerc Metab.* 2008;18(2):131-141.

169. Petrie HJ, Chown SE, Belfie LM, et al. Caffeine ingestion increases the insulin response to an oral-glucose-tolerance test in obese men before and after weight loss. *Am J Clin Nutr.* 2004;80(1):22-28.

170. Keijzers GB, De Galan BE, Tack CJ, Smits P. Caffeine can decrease insulin sensitivity in humans. *Diabetes Care.* 2002;25(2):364-369.

171. Greer F, Hudson R, Ross R, Graham T. Caffeine ingestion decreases glucose dis-posal during a hyperinsulinemic-euglycemic clamp in sedentary humans. *Diabetes.* 2001;50(10):2349-2354.

172. Graham TE, Sathasivam P, Rowland M, Marko N, Greer F, Battram D. Caffeine ingestion elevates plasma insulin response in humans during an oral glucose toler-ance test. *Can J Physiol Pharmacol.* 2001;79(7):559-565.

173. Thong FS, Graham TE. Caffeine-induced impairment of glucose tolerance is abolished by beta-adrenergic receptor blockade in humans. *J Appl Physiol.* 2002;92(6):2347-2352.

174. Thong FS, Derave W, Kiens B, et al. Caffeine-induced impairment of insulin action but not insulin signaling in human skeletal muscle is reduced by exercise. *Diabetes.* 2002;51(3):583-590.

175. Robinson LE, Savani S, Battram DS, McLaren DH, Sathasivam P, Graham TE. Caffeine ingestion before an oral glucose tolerance test impairs blood glucose man-agement in men with type 2 diabetes. *J Nutr.* 2004;134(10):2528-2533.

176. Johnston KL, Clifford MN, Morgan LM. Coffee acutely modifies gastrointestinal hormone secretion and glucose tolerance in humans: glycemic effects of chlorogenic acid and caffeine. *Am J Clin Nutr.* 2003;78(4):728-733.

177. Sachs M, Forster H. Effect of caffeine on various metabolic parameters in vivo. *Z Ernahrungswiss.* 1984;23(3):181-205.

178. Kiefer J. Modulated tissue response. *Carb Backloading.* 2012:16-20.

179. Brice CF, Smith AP. Effects of caffeine on mood and performance: a study of realistic consumption. *Psychopharmacology (Berl).* 2002164(2):188-192.

180. Greden JF. Anxiety or caffeinism: a diagnostic dilemma. *Am J Psychiatry.* 1974;131(10):1089-1092.

181. Stern KN, Chait LD, Johanson CE. Reinforcing and subjective effects of caffeine in normal human volunteers. *Psychopharmacology (Berl).* 1989;98(1):81-88.

182. Eaton WW, McLeod J. Consumption of coffee or tea and symptoms of anxiety. *Am J Public Health.* 1984;74(1):66-68.

183. Lee MA, Cameron OG, Greden JF. Anxiety and caffeine consumption in people with anxiety disorders. *Psychiatry Res.* 1985;15(3):211-217.

184. Rihs M, Muller C, Baumann P. Caffeine consumption in hospitalized psychiatric patients. *Eur Arch Psychiatry Clin Neurosci.* 1996;246(2):83-92.

185. Clegg DO, Reda DJ, Harris CL, et al. Glucosamine, chondroitin sulfate, and the two in combination for painful knee osteoarthritis. *N Engl J Med.* 2006;354(8):795-808.

186. Bausell RB. *Snake Oil Science: The Truth About Alternative and Complementary Medicine.* New York, NY: Oxford University Press; 2007:251.

187. Update on glucosamine for osteoarthritis. *Medical Letter.* 2001;43:111-112.

188. Product review: Glucosamine and Chondroitin. *ConsumerLab.* Accessed Jan 22, 2002.

189. Product review: Joint supplements (glucosamine, chondroitin, and MSM). *ConsumerLab.* Updated Sep 22, 2007.

190. Wackerhage H, Ratkevicius A. Signal transduction pathways that regulate muscle growth. *Essays Biochem.* 2008;44:99-108. Review.

191. Kimball SR, Jefferson LS. Signaling pathways and molecular mechanisms through which branched-chain amino acids mediate translational control of protein synthesis. *J Nutr.* 2006;136(1 Suppl):227S-231S. Review.

192. Hay N, Sonenberg N. Upstream and downstream of mTOR. *Genes Dev.* 2004;18(16):1926-1945. Review.

193. Borgenvik M, Apro W, Blomstrand E. Intake of branched-chain amino acids influences the levels of MAFbx mRNA and MuRF-1 total protein in resting and exercising human muscle. *Am J Physiol Endocrinol Metab.* 2012;302(5):E510-E521.

194. Pasiakos SM, McClung HL, McClung JP, et al. Leucine-enriched essential amino acid supplementation during moderate steady state exercise enhances postexercise muscle protein synthesis. *Am J Clin Nutr.* 2011;94(3):809-818.

195. Kiefer J. Leucine. *Carb Backloading.* 2012:96-98.

When an athlete has an orthopedic injury—damage to bone, ligament, tendon, or muscle—the last thought in a practitioner's mind is how to modify that athlete's diet to optimally heal from that injury. Typically, the practitioner is focused solely on the acute and physical aspects of the injury, mainly controlling inflammation, maintaining range of motion in minor injuries, and in some cases immobilizing joints for more potentially serious injuries. While the rehabilitation of the injury is beyond the scope of this text, it is worth understanding if it is possible to improve recovery and decrease lost time for an athlete with modifying their diet to be a catalyst during the recovery process.

The recovery and rejuvenation of an orthopedic injury is an ongoing process; therefore, optimizing nutrient intake would theoretically benefit the athlete, no matter what stage during the injury process they are in. Bone, tendon, ligament, and muscle differ in how quickly they can realistically remodel and recover, the biggest factor being blood flow to the affected area as well as the turnover rate of the tissue. The turnover rate is the rate at which the tissue building and breakdown occurs. If the injured tissue has a higher turnover rate, it can more rapidly rebuild strong tissue. Muscle has great blood flow and a comparatively high rate of turnover so it can heal quite rapidly. In contrast, tendons and ligaments have relatively poorer blood flow and tissue turnover and tend to heal much more slowly. Bone can be confusing because it is somewhere in the middle with decent blood flow and tissue turnover but a much larger structure, so the absolute turnover in bony tissue can take much longer to fully turnover.

In order to consult athletes properly on modifying their diet for injury recovery, we must first understand what happens at the cellular level, how best to adjust total calorie intake and adapt macronutrient ratios, and what potential supplements are available to assist during the recovery of the injury.

Eating Optimally for Injury Recovery

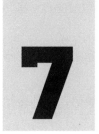

KEY TAKEAWAYS

* Prior to assessing dietary needs for orthopedic injury, practitioners must understand the injury process at the cellular level.
* Obtaining necessary protein intake while injured is much easier than most athletes think.
* Several potentially anti-inflammatory supplements can aid in recovery but should be properly vetted for efficacy.
* As important as consuming sufficient dietary fat is, consuming the right type of dietary fats may be equally as important.
* It is important to eat more anti-inflammatory foods, reduce carbohydrates, and potentially complement with certain supplements that may help recover faster.

WHAT HAPPENS DURING AN INJURY?

Once an orthopedic injury occurs, the first stage of recovery begins. That stage is called *inflammation*, followed by proliferation and remodeling. There is little that can be done to speed up physiology, but we can provide the optimal environment for healing or do the opposite and impair the process. We must understand these phases because even though they are discussed separately, they do overlap and sometimes are difficult to distinguish.

Amato D. *An Athletic Trainer's Guide
to Sports Nutrition (pp 113-122).*
© 2019 SLACK Incorporated.

The injury-healing process is actually very well automated and organized, even though the recipient of the injury may disagree with the amount of pain he or she may be in, but the body has very good strategies to heal itself. The process is very predictable.

Coagulation and Inflammation

The first phase of the healing process is coagulation, followed by inflammation. In an orthopedic injury, there will be bleeding and chemical mediators brought to the injury site to facilitate a "plugging of the dam" in order to prevent further injury. This is why the first line of defense is cryotherapy, usually combined with immobilization and compression. Since the body tends to overdo it with chemical mediators to the injured area, more inflammation than is necessary occurs at the injury site. When that happens, secondary cell death transpires due to hypoxia.[1] **Interstitial** fluid fills up space and occludes blood and lymph vessels, which prevents oxygen in the blood from getting to damaged tissue. Recently, arguments have been made against the use of ice; however, these claims are in the context of chronic injury or simple muscle damage from regular training when the inflammation response is much more subdued. In those contexts, the argument is perhaps valid. That is, of course, vastly different from typical acute orthopedic injuries that practitioners will see, and the physiological response described previously plainly shows the benefit of proper cryotherapy in response to an acute orthopedic injury.

Proliferation and Remodeling

While some degree of inflammation will be ongoing throughout the entire recovery process, eventually most of the inflammation will dispel and the body will enter into the proliferation phase. During this phase, scar tissue will form at the injury site in a scattered manner, almost cobweb-like in design. Once the proliferation phase has ended, the body will begin remodeling the tissue. Remodeling implies that less scar tissue will form in favor of the proper tissue to replace what has been injured. Unfortunately, weaker scar tissue remains so the injured area typically does not regain full strength from pre-injury, which is why it is so important to eat optimally during this phase while strengthening the muscles and connective tissue around the area in order to further protect it from re-injury.[1]

It is imperative to understand how best to control inflammation during the early stages of recovery, and how best to support that process nutritionally. NSAIDS such as ibuprofen or naproxen sodium can be helpful in the short term; however, the potential for misuse, overuse, and side effects like stomach ulcers may result with long-term use.[2] Some inflammation is important for ideal recovery, and once the primary inflammation from injury has resolved, it is more important to modulate rather than eliminate inflammation. With that in mind, a number of dietary supplements have been studied and found to the inflammatory process so that excessive inflammation is avoided. Some work better than others, such as fish oil. Other compounds will be discussed as well but may have a lesser overall effect.

SUPPLEMENTS TO AID IN INJURY RECOVERY

Fish Oil

The term *fish oil* refers to the 2 main fatty acids that are of benefit, namely eicosa-pentaenoic acid (EPA) and docosahexaenoic acid (DHA). Fish oil has been shown to greatly modulate excessive inflammation in the body by decreasing negative **inflammatory cytokines**. Studies have used doses ranging from 1.5 to 5 g of total EPA/DHA per day, but unfortunately, with the number of different fish oil brands available, it can be difficult to decide which is best. The majority come in pill form and can be very large and difficult to digest, especially if you require a higher dose and need to take up to 16 pills/day. There are also liquid products such as Very Finest Fish Oil (Carlson Labs), which can be used in water or other drinks and may be preferable by those who are not able or willing to take large handfuls of pills. Fatty fish such as salmon or mackerel can also be eaten as a source of fish oil, but well-formulated pills or liquid contain much more EPA and DHA than one could consume just by eating fatty fish.[3]

Curcumin/Turmeric

Curcumin is a compound found in turmeric, a member of the ginger family. It has been shown to have a variety of modulating effects on inflammation and many swear by its use. The effective dose is high at 400 to 600 mg 3 times/day. It may cause stomach upset with extended use and it should not be combined with either anticoagulant drugs or high doses of NSAIDs.

Bromelain

Bromelain is a compound found in fresh pineapple that has been found to have anti-inflammatory compounds, and it also acts as in the stomach to aid with protein breakdown. Numerous studies have examined the impact of bromelain on the treatment of arthritis and found it to be effective at doses ranging from 200 to 2000 mg/day. While fresh pineapple has been recommended as a source of bromelain, it is difficult to determine how much is actually present or whether it is effective, thus supplementation is probably a better course of action.

White Willow Bark

White willow bark is nothing more than a naturally occurring form of aspirin (that is, aspirin was a synthetically created version) that can have anti-inflammatory effects and might be considered. While similar to aspirin, its overall metabolism seems to be less problematic than the synthetic form in terms of risks or side effects. The effective dose is 220 to 260 mg/day.

Other Anti-Inflammatory Compounds

There are a number of other inflammatory compounds that seem to be less well-studied but which may have potential benefits.[4] This includes pycnogenol (100 to 200 mg/day), boswellia (300 to 500 mg twice/day), cat's claw (1000 mg root bark in 8 oz water), or capsaicin/chili pepper (dose unknown). While a compound called *resveratrol* has shown some benefit in animal studies, it is invariably via injection and the fact is that the absorption of resveratrol when taken orally by humans is near zero. The compounds mentioned previously (fish oils, turmeric/curcumin, bromelain, white willow bark) are probably the best choices. To both control and modulate inflammation, the previously mentioned supplements could be taken with food. Indicated doses are typically found on the food label but vary from manufacturer to manufacturer. Consult a qualified medical professional for proper dosages.

HOW TO MANAGE CALORIE INTAKE

An interesting facet of nutrition strategy is how to modify when injured. Other than the obvious change of potentially switching from 10+ hours per week of rigorous exercise to be being bed-ridden in some cases, there are some metabolic changes that happen, and with supplementation and proper strategy, there may a chance to enhance healing. I will examine macronutrients, both in relation to their roles in the body as well as what may change while recovering from an injury. Foremost is protein, found mostly in animal products. Unquestionably, vegetable sources of protein exist with beans and nuts being relatively high in protein per serving and some grains containing at least a modicum of protein; however, these are by and large not well metabolized, as seen in previous chapters regarding veganism. That makes it fairly difficult to reach an athletes' protein requirement on a daily basis. This is significant because adequate dietary protein is absolutely necessary for optimal injury recovery. It is also well-established that more protein than might be needed by sedentary individuals is required during injury recovery from surgery.[3]

Protein

Protein intakes ranging from 0.7 g/lb (1.5 g/kg) all the way up to 0.8 to 1.0 g/lb (2 to 2.2 g/kg) may be required in cases of complete immobilization to optimize recovery from injury.[4] The amalgamation of new tissue requires that the body have more building blocks and enzymes extant than what is required for the athlete to normally maintain their current muscle mass, so more protein (and, therefore, calories) is necessary. It is worth stating, however, that this is much easier than the typical athlete would think. Many of us, nutrition professionals included, are inherently very poor at estimating portion sizes in that we vastly underestimate in general. Oftentimes, athletes consume almost twice as much protein as would be necessary to just maintain muscle mass.[5]

Free amino acid (FAA) levels also need to be kept high throughout the day. The extracellular concentration of essential amino acids, or the FAA pool—along with other transcription factors—determines the growth rate of skeletal muscle. Maximum protein anabolism happens when FAA levels are elevated throughout the day.[6-8]

Maximum anti-catabolism is the salient point here. When skeletal muscle is in an anabolic state, the cellular apparatus does everything in its power to cultivate new muscle tissue, which includes the prevention of proteolysis—the breakdown of muscle tissue. Protein oxidation elevates during a resistance training workout, so high FAA levels prevent muscle breakdown except during that type of exercise. Regardless of FAA levels, muscles do not integrate new protein into the cell. Muscle growth occurs before and after resistance training, but not during. Keeping FAA levels high during the workout blunts proteolysis, preventing muscle degradation.[9] Along with keeping FAA levels elevated, skeletal muscle also needs signals that tell them how much or how little of those FAAs to incorporate into the cell. Insulin is the primary hormone signal that causes positive incorporation into muscle cells. One of the essential amino acids, leucine, is a positive signal as well. Myostatin does the opposite by causing muscle breakdown. All of the essential amino acids and several nonessential amino acids (other than leucine) do not stimulate protein deposit and retention beyond normal.[6] Leucine, however, acts independently to speed muscle growth. The mechanism of action is beyond the scope of this text because of the complicated steps and understanding of specific pathways, but it is of paramount importance to know the role that leucine plays in muscle growth and retention.

Insulin is relatively easy to stimulate, either from a carb bolus (about 30 g of fast-acting carbs) or a large protein portion (about 25 g of whey for example), but downregulating myostatin is difficult and may only be done by resistance training, and mostly in men at that. It is possible that creatine decreases myostatin levels, which may explain the accelerated rates of muscle growth when supplementing with creatine monohydrate, explained better in the chapter on the supplement.

It would be difficult to underestimate the importance of protein in an athlete's diet in general, but that point is underscored when an athlete is injured. The body changes down to the cellular level must be clarified and well understood by practitioners in order to be able to properly prescribe the ideal diet modifications that would help optimize recovery.

Fats

Dietary fats, an often underappreciated macronutrient, is responsible for the creation of hormones, transport of fat soluble vitamins, and a host of other processes in the body, especially during an injury. The term for fats while floating around in the bloodstream is *triglycerides* (3 fatty acids bound to a single glycerol molecule). Triglycerides are found in most protein-containing foods and animal products, but foods such as fruits and vegetables have basically none. Not unlike carbs, one of their primary roles is to provide energy to the body, although they are also involved in cell membrane structure and cell signaling. Consuming sufficient amounts of dietary fat is critical both in a general sense, but particularly when recovering from an injury. That should certainly not be seen as giving free reign to eat as much fat as possible, as foods such as nuts are incredibly easy to overeat and contain a very high amount of fat per serving.

As important as consuming sufficient dietary fat is, consuming the right type of dietary fats may be equally as important. The 3 primary classes are monounsaturated fats, polyunsaturated fats, and saturated fats. Monounsaturated fats are liquid at room temperature and constitute the majority of fat in most fat-containing foods, but they are most commonly associated with vegetable oils such as olive oil.

The polyunsaturated fats are also liquid at room temperature and can be separated into the omega-6 and omega-3 fatty acids. Omega-6 fatty acids are found in many foods, predominantly vegetable oils, chicken skins, and nuts. They are often found in excess in the modern American diet compared to omega-3s.

Saturated fats are solid at room temperature and are predominantly found in animal products, except for coconut oil. Dietary fat intake should likely be at moderate to higher levels due to a decreased need for carbs from lack of activity.

Being that fat is necessary for hormone creation, transport of nutrients, metabolizing fat-soluble vitamins, energy, and a host of other important functions required for healing, fat intake must not be ignored. On the other end of the spectrum, carbs are not necessary for energy requirements if the athlete is not exercising. Many carb-containing foods are **hyperpalatable**, less satiating, and, therefore, easier to overeat.[10] For those reasons, it is much easier and reasonable to shift to a higher fat/protein, lower carb diet while recovering from injury in order to prevent fat gain and optimize injury recovery.

Carbohydrates

Carbs are classified into simple and complex molecules. Simple carbs are monosaccharides and disaccharides. Those terms define how many carbon atoms they contain. Monosaccharides, therefore, have one carbon atom and disaccharides have two carbon atoms. They cannot be further hydrolyzed into simpler molecules and, for that reason, get broken down to either be stored as muscle glycogen or liver glycogen, used as energy, or converted into part of a triglyceride molecules to be stored into fat cells. Examples of monosaccharides are glucose, galactose, and fructose. Disaccharides are sucrose (glucose and fructose), lactose (galactose and glucose), and maltose (2 glucose bonds).

Complex carbs such as oligosaccharides or polysaccharides are ambiguously named by government nutrition professionals because foods that contain complex carbs typically also have indigestible fiber as well; however, they are more accurately named due to the number of sugar atoms in them. Oligosaccharides are molecules with 3 to 10 sugar atoms such as maltodextrin or corn syrup. Polysaccharides are longer chains of 10+ sugar atoms such as glycogen.

Simple and complex carbs also loosely correlate with the glycemic index. The glycemic index is a number associated with a particular food that indicates the food's effect on a person's blood sugar level. A value of 100 represents the foods that are an equivalent amount of pure glucose.[10]

While the glycemic index represents the total rise in a person's blood sugar level following consumption of the food, it may or may not represent the rapidity of the rise in blood sugar. The specific rise of blood sugar can be influenced by a host of other influences, such as the quantity of fat or protein eaten with the food. The gastroenterologist is useful for understanding how the body breaks down carbs[10] and only takes into account the available carbs in a food. The indigestible fiber that is in complex carbs travels all the way through to the large intestine where it gets fermented into short-chain fatty acids,[11] and thus has no effect on blood sugar.

Though the accuracy of the glycemic index is precise, it is largely irrelevant to humans because we typically do not eat singular foods in isolation. For instance, a mixed meal of a hamburger and fries may have a white bun and fries that are high on the glycemic index, but also contains beef that is high in fat and protein, both of which blunt the effect on a person's blood sugar, causing the overall glycemic index of the meal a moot point.

Starches like pasta, breads, rice, fruits, and many vegetables make up the majority of carb-heavy foods. Primarily, dietary carbs provide energy to the body, but the hormonal response to eating carbs creates an anabolic (tissue building) state in the body, which is critical for rebuilding and laying down new tissue, caused by the concomitant rise in insulin as a response. This response can be very beneficial when used sparingly to "challenge the system" and reset certain hormonal milieu such as that of leptin and ghrelin.[12] It can also be very detrimental if used multiple times per day like the typical American diet because excess energy gets converted to fat, and excess glucose in the blood stream will strain the pancreas.

Fruit and vegetables contain many nutrients that benefit overall health in general. Green vegetables like broccoli, green beans, or lettuce should ideally be part of every meal with good sources of animal protein such as grass-fed red meat or pork, with limited if any starchy carbs. Once the remodeling stage of recovery is well under way and the athlete is able to exercise (use excess glycogen stores), then increasing carb intake proportionate to activity is prudent.

Micronutrients

Micronutrients are described as vitamins and minerals, named because only small quantities are needed for survival. In addition to their other roles in the body, many are important in injury recovery. The majority of micronutrients have a recommended daily allowance, and ingesting more than that is at best not beneficial, and at worst dangerous.

Specific micronutrients that are critically involved in tissue repair are vitamin A, B vitamins, vitamin C, zinc, copper, and manganese, and deficiencies of these nutrients tends to be fairly rare, except in special cases like runners who eliminate red meat and end up sweating out zinc, thus becoming zinc-deficient. While all of these are involved in general injury healing, bone has additional nutrients including calcium, vitamin D, vitamin K, magnesium, silicon, and possibly boron, and all of these are often deficient in the modern diet.

CONCLUSION

It is important to eat more anti-inflammatory foods, reduce carbs, and potentially complement with certain supplements that may help recover faster. Eating healthy fats such as those from avocado, olive oil, mixed nuts and seeds, and fatty fish as well as ensuring a side of green vegetables is a reasonable basic recommendation to give athletes. Foods to avoid would be those that would increase excessive inflammation such as vegetable oils, trans fats (except for conjugated linoleic acid found in red meat), and excessive saturated fats, especially if still eating a lot of carbs.

Athletes need to eat enough when training and recovering. When you are injured and recovering, you should eat less than you did when you were training hard but more than you would if you were completely sedentary. There is a fine line and trial and error may take some getting used to for each individual.

At the 10,000 food view, practitioners may need to give only very basic recommendations to start out, depending on the individual needs of the athlete. Eating at least 1 g of protein per pound of lean body mass, balance dietary fats (and get more omega-3s than omega-6s), and eating a lot of vegetables with occasional fruit is a good starting point. Beyond that, many factors come into play and must be considered. Gender, type of athlete, food allergies or intolerances, preferences, and schedule all will shape the way an athlete can optimize his or her recovery.

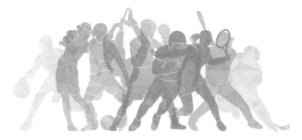

DEFINITIONS

Interstitial: The space in between cells and structures

Inflammatory cytokines: A type of signaling molecule that is excreted from immune cells like helper T-cells and macrophages, and certain other cell types that promote inflammation

Hyperpalatable: Non-nutritious food (ie, sugar, additives) that have artificially elevated flavors and suppress hypothalamic pituitary adrenal axis activity, impacting cortisol levels negatively

REFERENCES

1. Demling RH. Nutrition, anabolism, and the wound healing process: an overview. *Eplasty.* 2009;9:e9.
2. Morelli KM, Brown LB, Warren GL. Effect of NSAIDs on recovery from acute skeletal muscle injury: a systematic review and meta-analysis. *Am J Sports Med.* 2018;46(1):224-233.
3. Fusini F, Bisicchia S, Bottegoni C, Gigante A, Zanchini F, Busilacchi A. Nutraceutical supplement in the management of tendinopathies: a systematic review. *Muscles Ligaments Tendons J.* 2016;6(1):48-57.
4. Curtis L. Nutritional research may be useful in treating tendon injuries. *Nutrition.* 2016;32(6):617-619.
5. Buchholz AC, Schoeller DA. Is a calorie a calorie? *Am J Clin Nutr.* 2004;79(5): 899S-906S.
6. Millward DJ. Macronutrient intakes as determinants of dietary protein and amino acid adequacy. *J Nutr.* 2004;134(6 Suppl):1588S-1596S.
7. Munro HN. Energy and protein intakes as determinants of nitrogen balance. *Kidney Int.* 1978;14(4):313-316.
8. Edens NK, Gil KM, Elwyn DH. The effects of varying energy and nitrogen intake on nitrogen balance, body composition, and metabolic rate. *Clin Chest Med.* 1986;7(1):3-17.
9. Rand WM, Pellett PL, Young VR. Meta-analysis of nitrogen balance studies for estimating protein requirements in healthy adults. *Am J Clin Nutr.* 2003;77(1):109-127.

10. Glycemic Research Institute. Glycemic index testing. http://www.glycemic.com. Accessed October 5, 2017.
11. Randle PJ, Newsholme EA, Garland PB. Regulation of glucose uptake by muscle. 8. Effects of fatty acids, ketone bodies and pyruvate, and of alloxan-diabetes and starvation, on the uptake and metabolic fate of glucose in rat heart and diaphragm muscles. *Biochem J*. 1964;93;652-665.
12. Tipton KD. Nutritional support for exercise-induced injuries. *Sports Med*. 2015;45:93-104.

At some point during a practitioner's career, an athlete is going to inevitably ask, "When should I eat?" and "Is there an anabolic window after I work out to eat carbs? Protein?"

When athletes are attempting to make major physiological body changes such as increasing muscle mass, decreasing body fat, or improving energy, they tend to micromanage their own eating habits to get even a small edge over the next person. It is the job of the practitioner to understand which questions are worth answering and which are minutia that are not worth the athlete's time or effort.

The most important concept practitioners need to know is that of what the goal of the athlete is. To that end, does nutrient timing matter for performance, body composition, health, or muscle hypertrophy? Furthermore, the term *nutrient timing* often gets thrown around without a singular definition. For our purposes, it will be defined as eating specific nutrients at specific times in order to further a specific goal.

Understanding the term *nutrient timing* is paramount to learning the concepts around it. Two major components of nutrient timing have come to the forefront of the subject and will be discussed here. Recent research concerning the diurnal rhythm of certain hormones like cortisol, insulin sensitivity, adiponectin, and growth hormone have elucidated whether shifting calorie consumption (or even carbohydrate consumption) toward the later part of the day could be of benefit from a health standpoint. This research has dovetailed toward whether there is a "window" of opportunity to eat as it correlates with timing of resistance training exercise.

Nutrient Timing

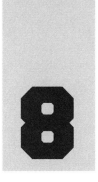

KEY TAKEAWAYS

* Nutrient timing is a complex subject that is widely debated, so practitioners would do well to understand the context on an individual basis.
* The majority of nutritional intervention studies are not comparing what subjects ate, but what they tell the investigators they ate.
* While total caloric load may be beneficial to shift toward the evening hours, it may be that it is more of a correlation and not necessarily the caloric load that makes a difference.
* There are a large number of parameters that can be measured to quantify the effectiveness of a certain diet plan that focuses on body fat reduction.
* Recommendations for eating on competition days differ between athletes depending on what energy system they primarily use during activity.

WILL SHIFTING CALORIE INTAKE TOWARD THE LATER PART OF THE DAY IMPROVE BODY COMPOSITION PARAMETERS?

Recent research has brought about several different diet strategies that employ an approach that shifts carbohydrates, calories, or both toward the later part of the

Amato D. *An Athletic Trainer's Guide to Sports Nutrition (pp 125-141).*
© 2019 SLACK Incorporated.

day, with varying degrees of results and efficacy. Many studies have been able to link energy regulation to the circadian rhythm in humans at the physiological and molecular levels,[1-4] emphasizing that the timing of food intake itself may play a significant role in weight regulation. Typical mixed meal weight loss protocols tend to fail long term because with food restriction come eating binges and emotional and cognitive disorders.[5-8] What practitioners need to figure out is the best way to feed obese people a **hypocaloric diet** where they are satiated, are compliant, and feel confident that they can stick to the regimen in order to facilitate long-term success.

An effective weight loss program is centered on modifications of diet, behavior, and physical activity, with the goal of promoting the loss of excess body fat and maintaining the appropriate amount of lean body mass that is necessary for optimal health and athletic performance.[9] Although restriction of caloric load is an effective means for reducing body weight, the role of specific dietary factors in maximizing the proportion of fat loss and minimizing the loss of muscle mass is less clear. Certain aspects of eating behavior, such as the time of day those meals are ingested, may have important consequences for weight control.

One hormone of many that is affected by eating behavior is leptin. Leptin has been described as the "information provider" of adipose tissue status to receptors in the brain. In short term, it contributes to regulation of hunger, satiety, and food intake[1-3] along with other hormones such as **adiponectin**, ghrelin, and cortisol. Previous studies have described a typical diurnal pattern of leptin secretion that falls during the day from 0800 to 1600 hours, reaching its lowest point at 1300 hours and increases from 1600 with a zenith at 0100 hours.[4,5] This hormone responsible for satiety is at its highest levels when individuals are sleeping.

Adiponectin is considered to be "the link between obesity, insulin resistance, and the metabolic syndrome."[10] Adiponectin plays a role in energy regulation as well as in lipid and carb metabolism, reducing serum glucose and lipids, improving insulin sensitivity, and having an anti-inflammatory effect by regulating inflammatory cytokines.[11] Adiponectin's diurnal secretion pattern has been described in obese individuals (particularly with abdominal obesity), as low throughout the day. In normal weight subjects or overweight subjects following weight loss, a general increase in adiponectin concentrations is detected as well as a rise in the diurnal pattern during the daytime.[12,13] Ghrelin also has a diurnal secretion, peaking about 2 hours after waking, while insulin level (in healthy humans) is related to exogenous carb and protein intake.[12,13]

Adipose tissue, one of the energy storage sites of the body, is an endocrine organ that synthesizes and secretes a variety of adipocytokines. This includes hormones that regulate hunger and satiety as well as those associated with the development of insulin resistance; metabolic syndrome; and inflammation such as adiponectin, leptin, ghrelin, and insulin.[14]

We will examine the findings in studies comparing different meal time regimens with the goal of fat loss, and how the diurnal secretion of hormones related to circadian rhythm are related to that meal timing in order to better understand how to formulate a quality fat loss diet for an overweight population attempting to improve health. Studies regarding athletes specifically are very limited and practitioners must have the ability to extrapolate information in order to assess athletes properly.

Review of Current Data

Different meal timing scenarios may affect fat loss outcomes in obese individuals. Results showing specific positive outcomes could enhance practitioners' abilities to formulate weight loss diets that would be easier to comply with in comparison to regular calorie-restricted protocols that have shown poor results.[7,8]

Meal timing and circadian rhythm hormones are applicable subject matter while probing for studies that meet appropriate criteria to display nutrient timing, with adult subjects having a body mass index of 30 or greater, eating at least 70% of their daily caloric load either in the morning hours or evening hours, with at least one other group doing the opposite and/or a control (Table 8-1).

Multiple studies with compelling data show differences in various health parameters; however, most of them were very short term and the results cannot be seen as final unless they can be replicated.[15]

Sofer et al[16] studied Israeli soldiers that had a control group and an experimental group. Both groups ate the same caloric load, but the experimental group ate the majority of their carbs and calories after 5 pm. The results showed that plasma adiponectin and leptin both increased in the experimental group that ate most of their carbs and calories at night.[13] The experimental group lost 1.75% more body fat on average compared to the control group (6.98% vs 5.13%). Previous studies with different diets reported that during weight loss, leptin concentrations decreased, satiety levels were reduced, food intake renewed, and a slow regain of body weight occurred,[17-19] but at the end of this study, the experimental diet group had a higher **hunger satiety score** (H-SSc) in comparison to baseline, meaning the experimental group felt more satiated than the control group.

Keim et al[20] studied 2 groups. In this experiment, participants alternated between two 6-week phases of the same diet, of which 70% of the daily caloric intake was eaten in the morning or evening, respectively. They found that their morning eating group lost more weight than the evening eating group.[20] Larger morning meals caused greater weight loss compared to evening meals, but the extra weight lost was in the form of muscle mass, an interesting statistic for practitioners as athletes who are looking to decrease overall body fat are very protective of holding on to muscle mass. Overall, the larger evening meals preserved muscle mass better (.25 kg vs 1.28 kg) and resulted in a greater loss in body fat percentage (2.52% vs 1.83%) by about 38% more compared to the morning eating group over a 6-week period, measured via **bio-electrical impedance**.

In the very first calorie-controlled study on meal timing from 1987 by Sensi and Capani, it was found that weight loss did not differ when participants ate their entire daily calorie intake in the morning (10 am), evening (6 pm), or spread out evenly through 3 meals.[21] The study lasted 15 days, and over 60% of total weight lost was from water weight. Methods of measuring body and body fat were not mentioned. Lipid oxidation was consistently higher in the PM-group, but there were no differences in cortisol levels, blood pressure, or resting energy expenditure between the groups.

Table 8-1

Summary of Research Regarding Shifting of Calorie Intake Toward Nighttime

AUTHOR AND YEAR	STUDY DESIGN	FINAL N	SEX	METHOD FOR CONTROLLING INTAKE	AGE GROUP (YEARS)	FACTORS ADJUSTED	LENGTH
Schlundt et al, 1992[23]	Experimental study	45	F	Sample menu program, diet journal	18 to 55	BMI > 30	12 weeks
Sofer et al, 2011[16]	Experimental study	78	B	Metabolic ward	25 to 55	BMI > 30	6 months
Keim et al, 1997[20]	Crossover study	10	F	Metabolic ward	23 to 39	Premenopausal, regular periods, BMI > 30	105 days
Sensi & Capani, 1987[21]	Experimental study	15	B	Metabolic ward	26 to 31	140% ideal body weight+	18 days
Nonino-Borges et al, 2007[22]	Experimental study	12	F	Metabolic ward	18 to 55	BMI > 40, no medications	18 days

(continued)

TABLE 8-1 (CONTINUED)

SUMMARY OF RESEARCH REGARDING SHIFTING OF CALORIE INTAKE TOWARD NIGHTTIME

WEIGHT LOSS OUTCOMES	FAT LOSS OUTCOMES	OTHER RELATED OUTCOMES
Non-breakfast group lost more weight compared to breakfast group (8.9 kg vs 6.2 kg)	Similar between groups	Resting metabolic rate decreased by 6% in both groups, subjects who normally ate breakfast and were in the non-breakfast group were less compliant (81% vs 60% at 6 months)
11.6 kg in experimental group, 9.06 kg in control group	6.98% in experimental group, 5.13% in control group	Increased adiponectin (143.5% of baseline vs 113.9%), high-density lipoprotein (114 mmol/L --> 140 mmol/L vs 110 mmol/L --> 126 mmol/L), H-SSc (128% of baseline vs 93.4%) in experimental group. Larger drop in blood glucose (5.1 mmol/L --> 4.71 mmol/L vs 4.85 --> 4.77), C-reactive protein (8.2 mg/l --> 3.9 mg/l vs 3.4 --> 2.2), leptin (68% of baseline vs 122% in control) and smaller reduction in 12-hour leptin concentration (79.4% of baseline vs 73.8%) in experimental group.
AM-centered eating group lost more weight compared to PM-centered eating group (3.9 kg vs 3.27 kg)	PM eating group lost more fat compared to AM-centered eating group (2.52% vs 1.83%)	PM-centered eating group lost less fat-free mass compared to AM-centered eating group (25 kg vs 1.28 kg)
Statistically insignificant	Not listed	Lipid oxidation higher in PM eating group (exact numbers not given)
Similar between groups	Similar between groups	Unchanged salivary cortisol levels

Using almost the exact same setup as the aforementioned study by Sensi and Capani in 1987,[21] it was found that splitting the daily calorie intake evenly into 5 meals consumed every other hour between 9 am and 8 pm, eating all calories in the morning (9 to 11 am), or in the evening (6 to 8 pm) did not affect weight loss via bio-electrical impedance, metabolic rate via indirect calorimetric measurement, or serum cortisol over the course of three 5-day periods.[22]

Schlundt et al[23] considered a 12-week study where participants were either consistent breakfast eaters or non-breakfast eaters, who were assigned a breakfast or non-breakfast diet (one-half of the breakfast eaters were in the breakfast eating group, and the other half were in a non-breakfast eating group; the same applied for those who were non-breakfast eaters). Caloric load was identical, but the breakfast group ate a breakfast meal in addition to 2 other meals, while the non-breakfast group shifted their calories to only 2 later meals. The non-breakfast eaters who continued without breakfast lost the least amount of weight (6.6 kg), while the breakfast eater group that was in the non-breakfast group lost the most weight (8.8 kg).[23] Both groups lost similar amounts of weight and body fat, but the non-breakfast groups showed better compliance rates at the follow-up 6 months later (81% vs 60%).

Data Extrapolation

Though the data show that the difference between morning and evening eating was not a large one, it was interesting that Sofer et al[16] showed statistically significant changes in leptin, adiponectin, ghrelin, and insulin sensitivity when humans shift calorie intake. Also of note is that Sofer et al[16] was the only study that specifically portioned carbs until nighttime in their experimental group.

Cortisol may not be affected by **chronobiology** as evidenced by Nonino-Borges et al[22] and Sensi and Capani,[21] but it is difficult to make that conclusion based on the study duration that only lasted 5 days and 18 days, respectively. It is plausible that cortisol is more affected by stress and sleep habits. The diurnal secretion of cortisol and the metabolic environment created by it at certain times of the day imply that there are more favorable patterns for eating calories and carbs throughout the day. It is difficult to elucidate those patterns due to the inconsistency of hormone recording in different studies. Accuracy, consistency, and thoroughness will help show more defining results in future studies.

Specific inclusion criteria for nutrient timing studies to ensure study data accuracy were adhered to because, oftentimes, nutritional intervention studies are not comparing what subjects ate, but what they tell the investigators they ate. That can lead to poor data and confusing results. Most studies used bio-electrical impedance to determine body fat analysis, but weight, waist size, and blood testing occurred as well with fewer margins for error. Some studies also used surveys from subjects to determine satiety and compliance, emphasizing the importance of those aspects of weight loss. This is important because of the variation of widespread practices and advice given to obese individuals in order to improve body composition. A further look into what we know about these hormones, circadian rhythm, and possible mechanisms may elucidate a more consistent and reliable way to reduce body fat rather than current practices that are difficult to comply to or have poor results.[7,8]

Schlundt et al[23] discovered that baseline breakfast skippers who were put on a breakfast diet got more favorable results than those who continued the breakfast-skipping pattern. In other words, going from skipping breakfast to eating breakfast showed a positive correlation for body weight control compared to those who skipped breakfast the entire time. This was an odd result because most favorable results in the study were with breakfast skipping amongst the "controlled" eaters (habitual breakfast eaters). The implication of these seemingly inconsistent findings might be related to other issues such as impulse control. Dysregulated eating habits, such as skipping breakfast when normally eating it, tends to go right along with uninhibited and impulsive eating.[24] Eating breakfast might therefore be of benefit for those with poor self-control in order to control ghrelin and leptin levels better.

The most interesting aspect of the Schlundt study[23] was that the breakfast eating groups showed a slight increase in depression-induced eating, whereas the subjects in the non-breakfast group showed a slight decrease. Furthermore, subjects in the breakfast group saw the diet as more restrictive than the non-breakfast group according to surveys within the study. Perhaps it was these favorable effects on their social life that also resulted in the non-breakfast groups showing superior compliance rates at follow-up 6 months later (81% vs 60%).

While Keim et al[20] did show superior lean tissue preservation in the nighttime eating group, the study was very limited as it was only 10 females and body fat was measured via total body electrical conductivity, which may not be very accurate, but becomes less accurate because the subjects were exercising at least 3 times per week and hydration levels can skew those results if measurements were taken at differing times with regard to exercise. Being hydrated or exercise-induced sweating may make those measurements inaccurate.[25] Given that the nighttime group consumed a greater percentage of their calorie intake post-workout, this study might simply show the benefits of nutrient timing, and not bigger PM meals. It is plausible that a similar study that eliminated exercise as a confounder and had a much larger sample size would have produced more persuasive results.

The most compelling data from Sofer et al[16] showed improvement in body composition parameters as well as blood lipids, waist circumference, 12-hour leptin levels, and H-SSc. These data show that, while total caloric load may be beneficial to shift toward the evening hours, it may be that it is more of a correlation and not necessarily the caloric load that made a difference. Several outcomes of the data sets are shown in Figure 8-1.

Future research investigations would lead toward carb restriction early in the day to distinguish between caloric load and insulin secretion as possible factors that led to the results in this study. In addition to the increase in body fat loss, the experimental group had much better satiety levels based on the H-SSc. This could be one of the more important results, being that satiety can be one of the biggest hurdles to overcome for an obese individual looking to lose body fat.

The same study also showed a much higher concentration of adiponectin the experimental group (that ate carbs only at night) compared to the control group. When insulin is low, adiponectin is high, but adiponectin also follows a diurnal pattern: low during nighttime, high during daytime (in normal weight individuals). In

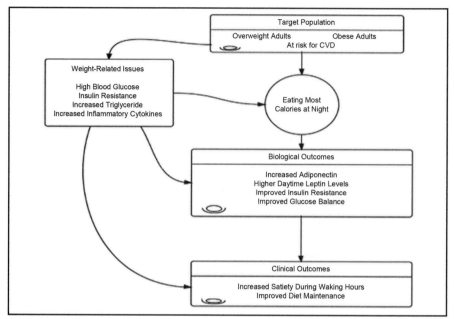

Figure 8-1. Evening eating fat loss mechanisms.

the obese, chronically high insulin causing chronically low adiponectin is a problem as it increases insulin resistance and inflammation.[10-13] By omitting carbs during the earlier part of the day, the researchers hypothesized that this would increase adiponectin and improve health markers more than the conventional diet.

As predicted, the big carb-rich dinner was able to alter leptin and adiponectin in a way that might have favored greater fullness and a better hormonal profile. The researchers stated, "The experimental diet modified daily leptin and adiponectin concentrations compared to those observed at baseline and to a control diet. A simple dietary manipulation of carb distribution appears to have additional benefits when compared to a conventional weight loss diet in individuals suffering from obesity."[13]

The changes in leptin and adiponectin in the Sofer study[16] bring up the possibility that other hormones with a diurnal secretion related to circadian rhythm may play a part in reducing body fat. The body releases ghrelin—the main hunger-control hormone[26]—in a pulsatile manner through the night with a peak occurring upon waking.[27-29] This spike incites hunger and is why some dieting subjects may not be able to adhere to a diet. Ghrelin also stimulates growth hormone release.[30,31] As growth hormone levels rise, the body releases more fat to be burned as fuel[32] and decreases the destruction of protein for use as fuel.[30] Growth hormone levels peak roughly 2 hours after waking if not eating earlier in the day.[33] Insulin sensitivity is also highest in the morning and drops throughout the day. That level will spike with the rise in blood sugar, kickstarting a downward spiral of fat burning, possibly hindering fat burning for the rest of the day.[34] While cortisol levels remain high, the insulin release causes new empty fat cells to be created.[35] The insulin also lowers levels of ghrelin and growth hormone.[27,33] These facts of human physiology imply that creating an insulin response during the first part of the day (especially for obese people) may inhibit fat loss results.

Summary

There are a large number of parameters that can be measured to quantify the effectiveness of a certain diet plan that focuses on body fat reduction. Calorie-controlled studies looking at the effects of distributing a fixed caloric load differently throughout the day are scarce. While short-term studies (15 to 18 days) do not find a statistically significant difference between early and late meal patterns, long-term studies (> 12 weeks) show that late eating patterns may produce superior results on body composition and/or diet adherence. This might be explained by more favorable nutrient partitioning after meals due to hormonal modulation.

The next phase of research may be to hold studies of a minimum of 12 weeks in a metabolic ward and record all relevant data for body composition parameters in both men and women. No single study compiled enough of all parameters to make a compelling conclusion. Shifting total calorie intake toward the evening may only have a correlation with preservation of lean tissue, increased satiety, and compliance and increased adiponectin levels, and it is paramount to define these mechanisms. It is plausible that since insulin and other hormones governed by circadian rhythm may play a large part in fat loss and satiety, we are overlooking how meal timing may affect those hormones.

When it comes to formulating a proper diet for an athlete based on his or her specific goals, practitioners must take all important aspects into consideration. This includes what time of day an athlete is eating, what macronutrients he or she is eating during different parts of the day and in what ratio, and how those habits effect performance and results. Individualization is key to learning how to optimize diet for health and performance.

IS THERE A POST-EXERCISE ANABOLIC WINDOW FOR FOOD?

Some practitioners say the most important aspect of nutrient timing research has been something we call the *post-workout anabolic window of opportunity*. The basic idea is that, after exercise, especially within the first 30 to 45 minutes or so, our muscles are more likely to uptake nutrients, and also that eating specifically protein and carbs is more beneficial before and after physical activity is more important than the absolute macronutrient intake for the day.

Recent data suggest that the total amount of protein and carbs you eat during the day is more important for body composition and performance than nutrient timing strategies.[36]

An intense resistance training workout results in the depletion of a significant proportion of stored fuels (including glycogen and amino acids) as well as causing damage to muscle fibers. Theoretically, consuming the proper ratio of nutrients during this time not only initiates the rebuilding of damaged tissue and restoration of energy reserves, but it does so in a super compensated fashion that enhances both body composition and exercise performance.[36]

One study even showed that waiting longer than 45 minutes after exercise for a meal would significantly diminish the benefits of training.[37] With these biological details thrust into athletes' minds, it became accepted that we should consume a fast-digesting protein and carb drink as soon as training ended, or potentially just prior to training a well. It became loosely apparent that the faster we could get these nutrients into our systems, the better.

Research regarding this impression has been all short term, and many studies show conflicting evidence even during a 1-week trial.[37] Even with that in mind, it is unclear whether any short-term benefit would lead into long-term results. In fact, recent longer-term studies, as well as 2 incredibly thorough reviews, indicate that the "anabolic window of opportunity" is actually a very open-ended period of time, much more so than most scientists used to believe.[36,38]

Muscle Glycogen Repletion

The question of enhancing muscle protein synthesis by timing protein intake is a separate subject than that of replenishing lost muscle glycogen through training, which is typically what athletes are more interested in. The theory would be that of performing intense physical exercise for extended periods, then replenishing that used up glycogen by eating large boluses of carbs in order to allocate energy stores for training the following day. This is most commonly known in the athlete world as the "pasta dinner."

The pasta dinner is a common tradition among team sports where the team get together the night before a big competition and eat large amounts of carbs, usually some type of pasta as the main course, in order to "carb up" for the next day's event. While the camaraderie and team-building aspect of the dinner can be advantageous, the food execution could be better.

Pasta is made from semolina flour, which is of course, purified wheat. Since we know from Chapter 2 that quick and high insulin spikes are more apt to shuttle glycogen into muscle cells to replenish storage than lower and longer insulin spikes, that gives us good information about what types of carbs are more beneficial for the purposes of restoring muscle glycogen for competition the following day. The ratio of how much amylose compared to amylopectin in carbs will help elucidate how quickly that food will be digested and what effect it has on insulin levels. Semolina flour is higher in amylose, making it a poor choice. It will cause a much lower rise in insulin that lasts a long time, which will upregulate the hormone lipoprotein lipase and actually make it more likely that the glucose sits around in the blood stream for long periods and becomes more likely to be shuttled into fat cells rather than muscle cells.

Carbs like rice have a ratio of 20:80 in favor of amylopectin, a carb that will cause a concomitant upregulation of hormone-sensitive lipase, a higher and shorter rise in insulin, and better replenishment of glycogen stores in muscle.

Carbs that athletes are better off consuming the night before competition are fast digesting, simple carbs. Complex carbs can be detrimental in terms of glycogen reple-tion. Examples of carb sources to include for the "pasta dinner" would be white bread, white rice, potatoes, and food sources made with those basic ingredients. This does not mean that eating junk food like cotton candy should be recommended. Many "sugar"-based candies are made from sucrose. Sucrose is a disaccharide that is com-posed of 50% glucose and 50% fructose. This fact is particularly important because fructose does not follow the same pathway for digestion as glucose and may hinder the wanted physiological response. Glucose-based foods should be at the forefront of the meal plan if glycogen repletion is the intended goal.

While eating large boluses of carbs the night before a competition and after some intense resistance training work is beneficial in terms of glycogen repletion, care must be taken to understand what types of carbs are more beneficial than others on a relative scale. Athletes are always trying to optimize their biological conditions when performing, so practitioners will need to explain this concept on an ongoing basis in order to dispel conventional wisdom, which is not correct.

TRAIN TO EAT AND EAT TO TRAIN

It would be impossible to make a blanket statement regarding what to eat dur-ing practice and competition days for all athletes because all athletes have different requirements in terms of energy systems during competitions. One way you can easily break down the differences would be sports that are repeat sprint sports that utilize glycolysis as the primary energy system, and also have competitions between 1 to 3 times per week (football, soccer, track sprinters, basketball, hockey, etc) and aerobic sports such as cross country, distance track runners, crew, etc. While much of the pre-competition recommendations may be similar, the most important differ-ence between the two are that the repeat sprint sport or strength sport athletes will burn through muscle glycogen much faster than the aerobic-based sports. This is due to the nature of the intensity of the activity. Repeated sprints utilize the anaerobic lac-tic, or glycolytic, energy system primarily. This literally means expending glycogen as energy. Aerobic-based sports' primary energy system used is the aerobic system. This system does not use one substrate exclusively, but rather bases its energy use on what is available. This is yet another reason why the "pasta dinner" for runners is especially not a valid way to improve performance during competition, and in many ways, can make athletes feel sluggish with low energy the following day.

RECOMMENDATIONS FOR
REPEAT SPRINT AND AEROBIC SPORTS

Due to the nature of this type of sport, more care should be taken to understand how an athlete feels on certain days. Since muscle glycogen can quickly get depleted through intense sprinting or repeated heavy lifting, a good indication of how much muscle glycogen an athlete has stored is how well he or she can actually repeat the same results from activity. If the athlete can normally perform ten 100-yard sprints for a time of 12 seconds, and on a specific day on repetition 5, his or her time is 16 seconds, you can bet that the muscle glycogen stores have been depleted and the athlete would need to replenish those after exercise.

Based on what we know about insulin and its interaction with certain hormones that have a diurnal rhythm, we can still only make limited generalizations because of the variation of each athlete, environment, schedule, habits, and sport. Likely, the most important concept is that of breakfast and, more specifically, the poor research surrounding breakfast and how that research is hindering performance.

Cortisol may be the most important hormone to understand, especially in the context of morning eating and morning training. When acting without elevated insulin levels and in a normal manner, cortisol triggers the breakdown of triglycerides into free fatty acids (FFAs) for metabolization a process known as **lipolysis**.[39,40] This takes into account someone who is not constantly stressed, which would cause chronically high cortisol levels or even reversed cortisol rhythms (low in the morning, high at night).

Morning time prior to eating is the one consistent time when insulin levels are very low and cortisol is high (assuming one is not diabetic), so cortisol accelerates fat burning in the morning if nothing interferes. Interference by triggering insulin release (through eating carbs) will not only shut down FFA mobilization at the time, but potentially throughout the entire day. This is important not just for athletes attempting to reduce body fat, but also for athletes whose main goal is to preserve muscle glycogen for training that day.

As we know fairly well now, insulin levels raise with the rise in blood sugar, beginning a decline in proper function: the early-morning release of insulin reduces fat burning for the entire rest of the day[41]; while cortisol levels remain high, the insulin release causes new empty fat cells to be created[7,21,35,42-47]; and the insulin lowers levels of ghrelin and growth hormone.[26,29,48,49]

Some practitioners may cite studies where students have better cognitive ability when they eat carbs at breakfast, or any breakfast at all; however, those studies were observations, and the students who did skip breakfast had another important variable—they were malnourished.[34,50-52] In fact, when kids skip breakfast, they behave and perform better cognitively throughout the entire school day.[7,21,34,46,47,50,51,53-57]

The overriding concept here is that, first thing in the morning, it is beneficial both for performance and health standpoints to keep insulin levels low, regardless of training schedule. If athletes are struggling during morning training and eating

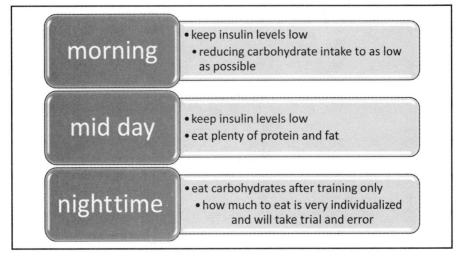

Figure 8-2. General guidelines for optimal glucose and energy control while training.

properly in the mornings, then they are not taking care to wake up with restored muscle glycogen from the previous night.

From morning on, we can extrapolate from what we know about muscle glycogen and adrenaline into training. Muscle glycogen is more available and muscles are more sensitive to adrenaline when insulin levels are low. When insulin levels in blood fall, glycogen synthesis in the liver diminishes and enzymes responsible for breakdown of glycogen become active. Glycogen breakdown is stimulated not only by the absence of insulin, but by the presence of glucagon, which is secreted when blood glucose levels fall below the normal range.[58] What this means is that pre-exercise sugar drinks or carb feedings are detrimental to performance, while at the same time very beneficial for recovery after activity is complete. A caveat to this would be intense exercise that lasts longer than approximately 2 hours. After that much training, it may be beneficial to add some fast-digesting carbs and electrolytes to continue training. Figure 8-2 gives a very generalized viewpoint for which a practitioner will need to individualize for each athlete.

CONCLUSION

Practitioners should hesitate to give blanket or general recommendations to any athlete without getting a full history of his or her situation. Though the salient points in this chapter apply to a large amount of the population, it is plausible that these recommendations will not work in certain circumstances. It has been referenced multiple times in this text that individualization is key, and often there will be a lot of trial and error when assessing and changing the eating habits of athletes. At the minimum, the well-researched facts here should be able to give practitioners a starting point with which to modify when making nutrition recommendations to athletes.

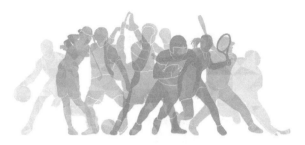

DEFINITIONS

Hypocaloric diet: A reduced-calorie meal plan

Adiponectin: A protein that is involved in regulating glucose levels as well as fatty acid breakdown

Hunger satiety score: A scoring system designed to quantify the effect different foods have on satiety

Bio-electrical impedance: A method for estimating body composition that determines the electrical impedance, or opposition to the flow of an electric current through body tissues, which can then be used to estimate total body water; this estimate can be used to estimate fat-free body mass and, by difference with body weight, body fat

Chronobiology: The branch of biology concerned with natural physiological rhythms and other cyclical phenomena

Lipolysis: The breakdown of fats and other lipids by hydrolysis to release fatty acids

REFERENCES

1. Ronti T, Lupattelli G, Mannarino E. The endocrine function of adipose tissue: an update. *Clin Endocrinol (Oxf).* 2006;64:355-365.
2. Klok MD, Jakobsdottir S, Drent ML. The role of leptin and ghrelin in the regulation of food intake and body weight in humans: a review. *Obes Rev.* 2007;8:21-34.
3. Picó C, Oliver P, Sánchez J, Palou A. Gastric leptin: a putative role in the short-term regulation of food intake. *Br J Nutr.* 2003;90:735-741.
4. Coleman RA, Herrmann TS. Nutritional regulation of leptin in humans. *Diabetologia.* 1999;42:639-646.
5. Ross CE. Overweight and depression. *J Health Soc Behav.* 1994;35:63-79.
6. Lopez KM. Value conflict: the level value conflict: the lived experiences of women in treatment for weight loss. *Health Care Women Int.* 1997;18:603-611.
7. Halberg F. Some aspects of the chronobiology of nutrition: more work is needed on "when to eat." *J Nutr.* 1989;119:333-343.
8. Howard B, Manson J, Stefanick M, et al. Low-fat dietary pattern and weight change over 7 years. *J Am Med Assoc.* 2006;295(1):94-95.

9.   American College of Sports Medicine. Proper and improper weight loss programs. *Med Sci Sports Exerc.* 1983;15:ix-xiii.

10. Gil-Campos M, Cañete RR, Gil A. Adiponectin, the missing link in insulin resistance and obesity. *Clin Nutr.* 2004;23:963-974.

11. Chandran M, Phillips SA, Ciaraldi T, Henry RR. Adiponectin: more than just another fat cell hormone? *Diabetes Care.* 2003;26:2442-2450.

12. Calvani M, Scarfone A, Granato L, et al. Restoration of adiponectin pulsatility in severely obese subjects after weight loss. *Diabetes.* 2004;53:939-947.

13. Yildiz BO, Suchard MA, Wong ML, McCann SM, Licinio J. Alterations in the dynamics of circulating ghrelin, adiponectin, and leptin in human obesity. *Proc Natl Acad Sci USA.* 2004;101:10434-10439.

14. Oishi K, Shirai H, Ishida N. Clock is involved in the circadian transactivation of peroxisome-proliferator-activated receptor alpha (PPARalpha) in mice. *Biochem J.* 2005;386:575-581.

15. Aragon AA, Schoenfeld BJ. Nutrient timing revisited: is there a post-exercise anabolic window? *J Int Soc Sports Nutr.* 2013;10(1):5.

16. Sofer S, Eliraz A, Kaplan S, et al. Greater weight loss and hormonal changes after 6 months diet with carbohydrates eaten mostly at night. *J Obes.* 2011;19:2006-2014.

17. Mars M, de Graaf C, de Groot LC, Kok FJ. Decreases in fasting leptin and insulin concentrations after acute energy restriction and subsequent compensation in food intake. *Am J Clin Nutr.* 2005;81:570-577.

18. Beck B, Richy S. Dietary modulation of ghrelin and leptin and gorging behavior after weight loss in the obese Zucker rat. *J Endocrinol.* 2009;202:29-34.

19. Ahima RS. Revisiting leptin's role in obesity and weight loss. *J Clin Invest.* 2008;118:2380-2383.

20. Keim N, Van Loan M, Horn W, et al. Weight loss is greater with consumption of large morning meals and fat-free mass is preserved with large evening meals in women on a controlled weight reduction regimen. *J Nutr.* 1997;127:75-82.

21. Sensi S, Capani F. Chronobiological aspects of weight loss in obesity: effects of different meal timing regimens. *Chronobiol Int.* 1987;2(4):251-261.

22. Nonino-Borges C, Borges R, Bavaresco M, et al. Influence of meal time on salivary circadian cortisol rhythms and weight loss in obese women. *J Nutrition.* 2007;23:385-391.

23. Schlundt DG, Hill JO, Sbrocco T, et al. The role of breakfast in the treatment of obesity. *Am J Clin Nutr.* 1992;55(3):645-651.

24. Brockmeyer T, Skunde M, Wu M, et al. Difficulties in emotion regulation across the spectrum of eating disorders. *Compr Psychiatry.* 2014;55(3):565-571.

25. Fuller NJ, Sawyer MB, Elia M. *Int J Obes Relat Metab Disord.* 1994;18(7):503-512.

26. Wren AM, Seal LJ, Cohen MA, et al. Ghrelin enhances appetite and increases food intake in humans. *J Clin Endocrinol Metab.* 2001;86(12):5992.

27. Natalucci G, Riedl S, Gleiss A, Zidek T, Frisch H. Spontaneous 24-h ghrelin secretion pattern in fasting subjects: maintenance of a meal-related pattern. *Eur J Endocrinol.* 2005;152(6):845-850.

28. Koutkia P, Canavan B, Breu J, Johnson ML, Grinspoon SK. Nocturnal ghrelin pulsatility and response to growth hormone secretagogues in healthy men. *Am J Physiol Endocrinol Metab.* 2004;287(3):E506-E512.

29. Shiiya T, Nakazato M, Mizuta M, et al. Plasma ghrelin levels in lean and obese humans and the effect of glucose on ghrelin secretion. *J Clin Endocrinol Metab.* 2002;87:240-244.

30. Moller L, Norrelund H, Jessen N, et al. Impact of growth hormone receptor blockade on substrate metabolism during fasting in healthy subjects. *J Clin Endocrinol Metab.* 2009;94(11):4524-4532.

31. Møller N, Schmitz O, Pørksen N, Møller J, Jørgensen JO. Dose-response studies on the metabolic effects of a growth hormone pulse in humans. *Metabolism.* 1992;41(2):172-175.

32. Nørrelund H, Møller N, Nair KS, Christiansen JS, Jørgensen JO. Continuation of growth hormone (GH) substitution during fasting in GH-deficient patients decreases urea excretion and conserves protein synthesis. *J Clin Endocrinol Metab.* 2001;86(7):3120-3129.

33. Salgin B, Marcovecchio ML, Humphreys SM, et al. Effects of prolonged fasting and sustained lipolysis on insulin secretion and insulin sensitivity in normal subjects. *Am J Physiol Endocrinol Metab.* 2009;296(3):E454-E461.

34. Martin A, Normand S, Sothier M, Peyrat J, Louche-Pelissier C, Laville M. Is advice for breakfast consumption justified? Results from a short-term dietary and metabolic experiment in young healthy men. *Br J Nutr.* 2000;84(3):337-344.

35. Hauner H, Schmid P, Pfeiffer EF. Glucocorticoids and insulin promote the differentiation of human adipocyte precursor cells into fat cells. *J Clin Endocrinol Metab.* 1987;64(4):832-835.

36. Schoenfeld BJ, Aragon AA, Krieger JW. The effect of protein timing on muscle strength and hypertrophy: a meta-analysis. *J Int Soc Sports Nutr.* 2013;10(1):53.

37. Cribb PJ, Hayes A. Effects of supplement timing and resistance exercise on skeletal muscle hypertrophy. *Med Sci Sports Exerc.* 2006;38(11):1918-1925.

38. Hoffman JR, Ratamess NA, Tranchina CP, Rashti SL, Kang J, Faigenbaum AD. Effect of protein-supplement timing on strength, power, and body-composition changes in resistance-trained men. *Int J Sport Nutr Exerc Metab.* 2009;19(2):172-185.

39. Baylor LS, Hackney AC. Resting thyroid and leptin hormone changes in women following intense, prolonged exercise training. *Eur J Appl Physiol.* 2003;88(4-5):480-484.

40. Tremblay A, Poehlman ET, Despres JP, Theriault G, Danforth E, Bouchard C. Endurance training with constant energy intake in identical twins: changes over time in energy expenditure and related hormones. *Metabolism.* 1997;46(5):499-503.

41. Hauner H, Entenmann G, Wabitsch M, et al. Promoting effect of glucocorticoids on the differentiation of human adipocyte precursor cells cultured in a chemically defined medium. *J Clin Invest.* 1989;84(5):1663-1670.

42. Ramsay TG, White ME, Wolverton CK. Glucocorticoids and the differentiation of porcine preadipocytes. *J Anim Sci.* 1989;67(9):2222-2229.

43. Bujalska IJ, Kumar S, Hewison M, Stewart PM. Differentiation of adipose stromal cells: the roles of glucocorticoids and 11beta-hydroxysteroid dehydrogenase. *Endocrinology.* 1999;140(7):3188-3196.

44. Nougues J, Reyne Y, Barenton B, Chery T, Garandel V, Soriano J. Differentiation of adipocyte precursors in a serum-free medium is influenced by glucocorticoids and endogenously produced insulin-like growth factor-I. *Int J Obes Relat Metab Disord.* 1993;17(3):159-167.

45. Suryawan A, Swanson LV, Hu CY. Insulin and hydrocortisone, but not triiodothyronine, are required for the differentiation of pig preadipocytes in primary culture. *J Anim Sci.* 1997;75(1):105-111.

46. Hirsh E, Halberg F, Goetz FC, et al. Body weight change during 1 week on a single daily 2000-calorie meal consumed as breakfast (B) or dinner (D). *Chronobiologia.* 1975;2(suppl 1):31-32.

47. Jacobs H, Thompson M, Halberg E, et al. Relative body weight loss on limited free-choice meal consumed as breakfast rather than as dinner. *Chronobiologia.* 1975;2(suppl 1):33.

48. Kojima M, Hosoda H, Date Y, Nakazato M, Matsuo H, Kangawa K. Ghrelin is a growth-hormone-releasing acylated peptide from stomach. *Nature.* 1999;402(6762):656-660.

49. De Bock K, Richter EA, Russell AP, et al. Exercise in the fasted state facilitates fibre type-specific intramyocellular lipid breakdown and stimulates glycogen resynthesis in humans. *J Physiol.* 2005;564(Pt 2):649-660.

50. Lopez-Sobaler AM, Ortega RM, Quintas ME, Navia B, Requejo AM. Relationship between habitual breakfast and intellectual performance (logical reasoning) in well-nourished schoolchildren of Madrid (Spain). *Eur J Clin Nutr.* 2003;57(Suppl 1):S49-S53.

51. Cueto S. Breakfast and performance. *Public Health Nutr.* 2001;4(6A):1429-1431.

52. Vaisman N, Voet H, Akivis A, Vakil E. Effect of breakfast timing on the cognitive functions of elementary school students. *Arch Pediatr Adolesc Med.* 1996;150(10):1089-1092.

53. Chandler AM, Walker SP, Connolly K, Grantham-McGregor SM. School breakfast improves verbal fluency in undernourished Jamaican children. *J Nutr.* 1995;125(4):894-900.

54. Pollitt E, Jacoby E, Cueto S. School breakfast and cognition among nutritionally at-risk children in the Peruvian Andes. *Nutr Rev.* 1996;54(4 Pt 2):S22-S26.

55. Lopez I, de Andraca I, Perales CG, Heresi E, Castillo M, Colombo M. Breakfast omission and cognitive performance of normal, wasted and stunted schoolchildren. *Eur J Clin Nutr.* 1993;47(8):533-542.

56. Simeon DT, Grantham-McGregor S. Effects of missing breakfast on the cognitive functions of school children of differing nutritional status. *Am J Clin Nutr.* 1989;49(4):646-653.

57. Dickie NH, Bender AE. Breakfast and performance in school children. *Br J Nutr.* 1982;48(3):483-496.

58. Costill DL, Coyle E, Dalsky G, et al. Effects of elevated plasma FFA and insulin on muscle glycogen usage during exercise. *J Appl Physiol.* 1977;43(4):695-699.

It is only a matter of time before a health care practitioner encounters an athlete with a special situation. Many physical special situations will require an assessment and specific instructions from a qualified physician and hospital-based Registered Dietitian, but there are several common physical issues that may come up that occasionally athletes feel more comfortable talking to an athletic trainer or therapist about. The most common of those ailments are eating disorders, food allergies, and diabetes.

While many of these athletes will already be under direct care for their specific ailment, some will not be and may depend on a trusted practitioner who sees them daily or weekly to give them proper advice. Each diagnosis discussed in this chapter has a clear physical manifestation, but it is important to understand that there is a strong mental component as well.

Even though changing your outlook will not cure diabetes, having diabetes can give you a poor outlook on sports and life. It is therefore of paramount importance to learn how to empathize with athletes and listen to their concerns while also not forcing them into doing something they may not understand. The most valuable aspect of these issues is to first educate yourself on the various ways to help the athlete, and let them choose for themselves what pathway they want to take.

Special Situations

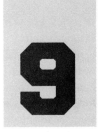

KEY TAKEAWAYS

* Incidence of reported food allergies as compared to positive tests for food allergies vary widely.
* There is an immense difference between a food allergy and a food sensitivity.
* Resistance training has a positive effect on treating symptoms of type II diabetes.
* Treatment of athletes with type I diabetes will differ from that of type II athletes.
* Lifestyle optimization is the best treatment for either form of diabetes.

FOOD ALLERGIES

Food allergies and sensitivities are becoming more common, not because more people get them, but we are now much more aware of the issues that can arise from some foods. Roughly 2 children in every classroom now have food allergies, which can be serious and potentially life-threatening.

When you do not have the necessary enzymes to digest or process certain foods, undigested irritants enter the large intestine and feed the bacteria that live there. This forces an overreactive inflammatory response and leads to the allergic reaction. This immune response is set from the foods we eat. It is through this progression of allowing undigested irritants to enter the large intestine to feed the bad bacteria, prompt inflammation, and then overstimulate the immune system that leads to food

Amato D. *An Athletic Trainer's Guide to Sports Nutrition (pp 143-157).*
© 2019 SLACK Incorporated.

allergies. These irritants can be anything from undigested carbohydrates, gluten, or casein protein.

Even if an athlete has been diagnosed by tests to confirm an allergy or sensitivity, or they have ruled out eating certain foods because they are more aware of negative reactions to them such as bloating, cramps, rash, hives, or the like, avoiding these foods forever is not a practical or enjoyable solution, especially if you travel with a team or for business often. A more practical solution would be to create a healthier intestinal environment by eating foods that feed the good bacteria in your gut such as kimchi, sauerkraut, or kefir. Probiotic (good bacteria) and prebiotics (food for good bacteria) supplements can be another avenue as well; however, the variations between what strains, quantities, combinations, and even shipping methods can be cumbersome for an athlete to decipher.

We know that food intolerances and allergies are largely caused by an overly sensitive immune response, and it has been shown that many factors influence your body's response to the food you eat. Lower rates of allergies are observed in children who have pets,[1] live on farms,[2] drink raw milk,[3] use fewer antibiotics,[4] are delivered via non-caesarean birth,[5] and are breastfed rather than bottle-fed.[6] In other words, children who have greater exposure to bacteria have an easier time dealing with them.[7]

Over the past decade or so, researchers have been able to show a number of mechanisms that cause allergic reactions to food. The body produces antibodies that leave traces we can test to detect potential allergies. You will see **immunoglobulin** A and E (IgA and IgE, respectively), with IgE being the predominant marker used to detect an allergy. Doctors can also look at any irregularities by performing a biopsy of the 2 sections of the digestive tract that connect the stomach to the small intestines. These pathways, along with experimenting with different dieting scenarios, can tell us whether certain foods actually do trigger allergies in an athlete.

Prior to this, we relied on guesswork and people's predetermined ideas by giving them a questionnaire with simple questions regarding whether they thought they had allergies to certain foods, such as "Do you have an allergy to milk? Yes or no?" Bloodwork and other current allergy testing are obviously much better. The problem is it is very difficult to change someone's mind without specific evidence. The following chart compares common foods that people "think" they are allergic to compared to what objective allergy testing tells us they are actually allergic to (Figure 9-1).[8-10]

The list of actual rates of food allergies among people comes from using a double-blind, placebo food challenge, and IgE detection procedure (the gold standard for detecting food allergies).[9,11-17] The disparity between the 2 columns in the picture show a clear difference between what people can believe and what is reality, and goes to show how powerful the placebo effect can be.

To be fair, if an athlete complains of symptoms consistent with food allergies, the practitioner should always investigate to try to find a cause instead of playing it off as something the athlete is making up. Other than anaphylactic shock from a severe allergy, athletes can have symptoms such as bloating, diarrhea, gas, acne,

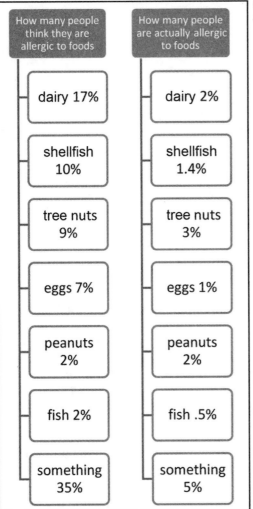

Figure 9-1. Comparison of perceived food allergy prevalence vs actual data.

unexplained rashes, fatigue, unexplained weight gain, and brain fog.[18] In many cases, athletes have no idea they have an allergy to a certain food until they stop eating it for a long enough period and the symptoms of that allergy subside.

Many people in general think they have a good allergy, and a considerable percentage of those people do not. With that in mind, it is prudent to err on the side of caution and investigate any correlation between foods and allergic reactions to them.

DIABETES

by Karl Nadolsky, DO

Introduction and Definition

Diabetes mellitus (DM) is a term describing a broad spectrum of disorders related to abnormal glucose (blood sugar) metabolism all sharing the common criteria of hyperglycemia (high blood sugar). Historically, "diabetes" refers to an increase in urine output, while "mellitus" refers to the "sweet" component of urine in DM because of hyperglycemia and ultimately glycosuria. The different types of DM represent an array of complex pathophysiologic disorders whereby hyperglycemia results from impaired or absent insulin secretion, varying degrees of resistance to insulin or "insulin resistance" (IR), and involving several other organ systems that work together harmoniously when intact.[19-21] Physical activity and exercise prescription are critical in the care for all patients with DM no matter which type, but appropriate understanding and clinical monitoring are essential for the safety and efficacy of implementation.[22-24]

Normal physiology of carb or glucose metabolism relies on the secretion of insulin, a peptide hormone, from the pancreatic beta cells in response to blood glucose levels or dietary consumption of carbs, protein, and even fat. The "first phase" is a rapid response of insulin secretion to blood glucose, which is followed by a "second phase" if necessary. Blood glucose taken up by GLUT2 transporters in the pancreas directly stimulates insulin. There are many complex pathways involved in this process, but they are beyond the scope of this chapter. Other specific components of receptors, transporters, and nuclear components of pancreatic beta cells play important roles and become clinically notable when mutated and underlie some of the rare genetic causes of DM, which will be briefly mentioned. Insulin secretion is also modulated by several other important sites, including incretin peptide hormone **secretagogues** from the intestine cells, complex hypothalamic control, and nervous system (vagal influence). Response to insulin is the ultimate uptake of glucose from the blood into muscle and/or fat via GLUT4 translocators. Physiologic response to exercise is insulin-independent uptake into muscle cells, which lowers blood glucose levels, decreasing insulin secretion and increasing counterregulatory hormones (glucagon and possibly catecholamines, growth hormone, and cortisol) to increase glycogenolysis/gluconeogenesis in the liver and lipolysis. With prolonged exercise, glucose uptake actually declines while the muscles increase utilization of free fatty acids.[19-22]

Pathophysiologically, hyperglycemia eventually can result from primary destruction of pancreatic beta-cells (which is also the "final common denominator") or a complex interplay of dysfunction IR from visceral/hepatic adiposity (obesity), muscular adiposity, dysfunctional neuroendocrine regulation from the hypothalamus, abnormal gut microbiome, and paradoxically increased glucose reabsorption from the kidneys amongst other pathways. This has been coined the "Egregious Eleven."[20]

Ultimately, the short-term complications of severe hyperglycemia (diabetic ketoacidosis, hyperosmolar state) and hypoglycemia along with the long-term complications including atherosclerotic macrovascular disease, microvascular disease (leading cause of blindness, kidney disease, etc), and nerve disease are the clinical indications for prioritizing comprehensive and holistic treatment of DM.

Classification of Diabetes Mellitus

As previously mentioned, there are different types and etiologies of DM corresponding to different aspects of that "egregious eleven" with the eventual result being pancreatic beta-cell failure and hyperglycemia usually at risk of the complications noted.

Type I DM (T1DM) is basically a primary pancreatic failure to secrete insulin due to autoimmune destruction of the ß-cells. Historically thought of as "juvenile" diabetes, it can occur at any age (older adults may develop latent autoimmune diabetes of adulthood) and is influenced by genetics and possibly environmental triggers. Insulin replacement therapy is absolutely necessary in these patients while risk of hypoglycemia and prevention is of utter importance (Table 9-1).

Type II DM (T2DM) basically develops on a foundation of complex genetic traits, obesity leading to IR/metabolic syndrome, and, finally, pancreatic failure with varying degrees of insulin insufficiency.

Both T1DM and T2DM are variably progressive and heterogeneous and may also be classified based upon their status of autoimmunity and insulin secreting ability.

Other forms of DM include gestational, neonatal, monogenic forms of DM, secondary DM (trauma, pancreatitis, etc), **endocrinopathies**, and other rare genetic defects or syndromes that are beyond the scope of this chapter.[21]

Diagnosis

Screening for diagnosis of diabetes may be conducted by physicians or other components of a health care delivery team upon patient presentation with acute symptoms of hyperglycemia or via routine screening for those at risk based upon obesity, age, and other associated factors. Screening and diagnostic tests include fasting plasma glucose, 2-hour plasma glucose following a standardized 75 gm glucose load (oral glucose tolerance test), or a hemoglobin A1c (HbA1c measures the glycation of red blood cells correlating to average blood glucose over their lifespan generally about 3 months).

Athletic trainers and exercise professionals should be aware of symptoms to feel comfortable referring to a higher level of evaluation and care. Classic symptoms of hyperglycemia in children and young adults with T1DM include fatigue, weight loss, blurred vision, and polyuria and polydipsia (increased urination and thirst/drinking, respectively). Those same symptoms can present in those with T2DM if they develop significant hyperglycemia before screening leads to diagnosis. Before hyperglycemia develops, IR may be considered if acanthosis nigricans is noticed. Acanthosis nigricans appears as velvety dark areas of skin, commonly the neck or axilla.

TABLE 9-1

CURRENT EXERCISE GUIDELINES FOR ADULTS WITH TYPE 1 DIABETES IN THE ABSENCE OF CONTRAINDICATION

	AMERICAN DIABETES ASSOCIATION	AMERICAN COLLEGE OF SPORTS MEDICINE	SOCIEDADE BRASILEIRA DE DIABETES	EUROPEAN ASSOCIATION FOR THE STUDY OF DIABETES	CANADIAN DIABETES ASSOCIATION
Frequency (days/week)	≥3 (aerobic)[1] and ≥2 (strength)	3 to 7[1]	≥3[1] and 2 to 3 (strength)	No recommendations	≥5
Type of Training	Aerobic or strength	Aerobic, strength, or combined	Aerobic, strength, or combined	Aerobic, strength, or combined	Aerobic, strength, or combined
Intensity	Moderate[2]	Moderate-vigorous[3]	Moderate-vigorous[5]	Moderate-vigorous	Moderate-vigorous[6]
Total Weekly Duration (minutes)	≥150	≥150[4]	≥150 (moderate) or ≥75 (vigorous)	≥150	≥150

1: With no more than 2 consecutive days without exercises

2: Aerobic at 50% to 70% of maximum heart rate (HR_{max})

3: Aerobic at 40% to 60% or at ≥60% of maximum amount of oxygen

4: Bouts of at least 10 minutes can be spread throughout the week

5: Aerobic at 50% to 70% or at >70% of HR_{max}

6: Aerobic at 50% to 69% or at 70% to 85% of HR_{max}. Strength exercises at 50% to 74% or at 75% to 85% of one repetition maximum.

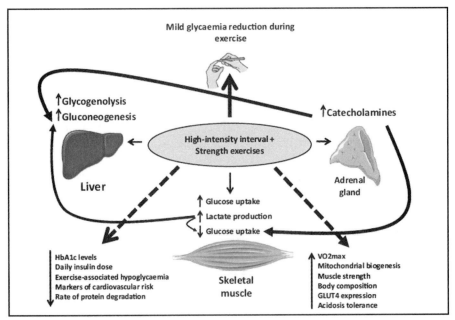

Figure 9-2. Suggested exercise training protocol for people with T1DM.

Diagnosis of T1DM now includes 3 stages. Stage 1 is those at risk due to positive autoimmunity but have no impaired glucose tolerance or impaired fasting glucose (IFG) and remain asymptomatic. Stage 2 criteria includes IFG (100 to 125 mg/dL; 5.6 to 6.9 mmol/L), 2-hour PG 140 to 199 mg/dL (7.8 to 11 mmol/L), or HbA1c 5.7% to 6.4% (39 to 47 mmol/mol). Stage 3 would be the classic criteria for diagnosis of DM, in the case of T1DM including autoimmunity, clinical symptoms, and glycemic criteria of FBG ≥ 126 mg/dL (7 mmol/L), 2-hour PG ≥ 200 mg/dL (11.1 mmol/L) or HbA1c ≥ 6.5% (48 mmol/mol).

T2DM is similarly diagnosed, but without evidence for autoimmunity. Essentially, all adults with clinical obesity (body mass index ≥ 25 kg/m^2 or ≥ 23 kg/m^2 in Asian ethnicities consistent with excess adiposity on exam) should be screened and everyone starting at age 45 years. Further monitoring and screening is beyond the scope of this chapter but can be reviewed via the American Diabetes Association (ADA) Standards of Care or American Association of Clinical Endocrinologists (AACE) clinical practice guideline for developing a DM comprehensive care plan (Figure 9-2).[21-23,25-27]

Management

While lifestyle optimization is the foundation for all patients with DM, for patients with T1DM, insulin replacement is the critical therapy needed as deficiency/absence is obviously the primary defect in their hyperglycemia. Most patients need to be treated with either multiple daily injections (MDI) to provide basal insulin (which basically covers the fasting state) and prandial insulin (to cover meals) or continuous subcutaneous insulin infusion (CSII or insulin pump). The basic goal is to keep blood glucose near a normal range with minimal fluctuations and, perhaps most importantly, avoid hypoglycemia. Other endocrine components of glycemic control (like glucagon) are dysfunctional in T1DM thus are at a very high risk of hypoglycemia. Some patients with T1DM will use a set amount of prandial insulin along with a "correction factor," which adds insulin if the blood glucose is higher than the goal going into a meal. Most patients with T1DM will utilize carb counting (and some the even more complex fat/protein counting) to calculate their bolus insulin needs in addition to a correction factor using either MDI or CSII. We are now to the point where one insulin pump on the market is coined a "hybrid closed-loop" as it uses a continuous glucose monitor with an algorithm to adjust the insulin dosing frequently to keep the blood glucose near its goal, which decreases overall hyperglycemia and hypoglycemia significantly. Patients with T1DM (and those with T2DM requiring basal/bolus insulin) need to monitor their glucose levels several times per day either by using glucose meters (self-monitoring blood glucose [SMBG] or a continuous glucose monitor [CGM]). Knowing these levels help patients and caregivers use the correct amount of insulin, eat accordingly, and exercise safely. Glycemic goals for everyone are personalized. HbA1c, representing chronic glycemia, should often be under 7%, but that goal may be lower for some and higher for others depending on their risk for hypoglycemia and other medical factors that influence the long-term microvascular and macrovascular outcomes. The ADA recommends pre-meal capillary plasma glucose about 80 to 130 mg/dL (4.4 to 7.2 mmol/L) and/or peak postprandial glucose <180 mg/d/L (10 mmol/L). These are also to be personalized based on several patient characteristics and minimizing the risk of hypoglycemia while optimizing glucose as low as is reasonably safe and stable. Glycemic goals for exercise and sport will be discussed later in this chapter.

For patients with T2DM, lifestyle and weight loss are the critical focus of therapy, often adjunctively treated with several classes of medications that work on areas of the "egregious eleven." Glucose goals are similar but have more factors as not all patients will be treated with insulin or drugs that increase insulin and thus are at much lower risk of hypoglycemia and generally have many other chronic conditions. Much of the chronic disease burden is due to obesity-related complications, like T2DM itself, metabolic syndrome, obstructive sleep apnea, established atherosclerotic cardiovascular disease, female reproductive disorders or male hypogonadism, liver disease, and arthritis to name a few.[28] AACE also suggests personalized glycemic goals for patients with T2DM, though it leans more aggressively toward "normal" levels for younger and otherwise healthier patients, including HbA1c <6.5%, pre-meal glucose <110, and 2-hour post-meal glucose <140. The types of medications used for these patients along with success of obesity treatment and optimization of lifestyle therapy may warrant lower personal goals. Knowing a little bit about the medications that patients may be taking could be important for athletic trainers to know when prescribing exercise (Table 9-2).

TABLE 9-2			
TYPE II DIABETES MELLITUS MEDICATION BASICS			
DRUG CLASS	**EXAMPLE**	**HYPOGLYCEMIA RISK***	**OTHER RISKS**
Biguinides	Metformin	No	Minimal
Sulfonylureas	Glimeperide	Yes	Minimal beyond hypoglycemia
DPP4 inhibitors	Sitagliptin	No	Heart failure
SGLT-2 inhibitors	Empagliflozin	No	Hypovolemia/ acute kidney injury
GLP-1 agonists	Liraglutide	No	Minimal
Thiazolidinedione	Pioglitazone	No	Fluid retention
A-glucosidase inhibitors	Acarbose	No	Minimal
*Medications may amplify risk of hypoglycemia when combined with insulin or sulfonylureas			

PHYSICAL ACTIVITY AND
EXERCISE PRESCRIPTION FOR ATHLETICS

Physical activity and exercise prescription for patients with T2DM is of utmost importance and arguably even more important in "prediabetes" and/or metabolic syndrome for intensive efforts to prevent the progression to overt diabetes. Glycemic control improves significantly through physical activity along and when combined with nutritional therapy and energy deficiency for weight loss, and it is a very powerful interventional tool (and preventive tool). A combination of aerobic and resistance training is recommended by all major diabetes-related practice guidelines.[22-26] Independently of insulin, exercise increases the uptake of glucose into muscle via GLUT4 transporters and improves insulin sensitivity up to 48 hours. In addition to glycemic improvements, aerobic exercise, resistance training, and "non-exercise activity" improve nearly all CVD risk factors and improve functional capacity along with well-being. Both the AACE clinical practice guideline on developing a comprehensive plan for T2DM and ADA standards of care recommend a minimum basic prescription of ≥150 min/week of at least "moderate-intensity" exercise using examples such as brisk walking, water aerobics, recreational play, etc. It is suggested to spread that over at least 3 days/week with no more than 2 consecutive days without activity. Progressive increasing in intensity and volume improves benefits and it is noted that high-intensity interval training at sufficient volumes (> 75 min/week) may be sufficient if physically able, and there are data to suggest it may even be better than continuous training for improving adiposity and glucose homeostasis.

Resistance training, incorporating all major muscle groups, is recommended to be prescribed 2 to 3 days/week. Achieving the goal of improved glycemic control and cardiometabolic improvements with resistance training can be accomplished in a variety of ways to be personalized for each patient. Higher volumes and progressive weights/intensity are more beneficial than using high weights and low repetitions. This could come in the form of nearly daily weight training focusing on one muscle-movement group and short rest periods (1 to 2 minutes) between sets of pushing to (or close to) failure or could be 2 to 3 days of full-body circuit training. Different types of free weights vs machines will need to be of careful consideration when prescribing a personalized program for individuals with T2DM.

An important point to emphasize for everyone—but especially patients at risk of or with T2DM—physical activity and exercise is beneficial at any amount or type of activity. Specific recommendations and goals are less important to split hairs over and encouraging the patients to do whatever they enjoy doing with increasing intensity and volume will be extremely beneficial.

For patients with T1DM, cardiometabolic and other long-term benefits are also important, but more attention and care must be paid to the acute bouts of exercise and monitoring post-exercise due to the heightened risk of hypoglycemia. During exercise, muscles utilize the available glucose in the muscle before turning to convert the muscular glycogen to glucose. Due to the enzymatic pathways, however, muscular glucose cannot prevent hypoglycemia. As noted previously, muscles uptake glucose independently of insulin, but glucose is certainly amplified in the presence of insulin. Compared to patients with T2DM, there is then an increased risk of hypoglycemia as the blood concentration of insulin is most often set and not under control of the pancreas, which would decrease secretion if functional. Increased blood flow to subcutaneous fat tissue (site of insulin injections) secondary to exercise may also elevate levels of insulin. Fear of hypoglycemia is one of the foremost barriers to initiating exercise, thus potentially missing out on the benefits. This problem is beginning to be mitigated by the first recently available hybrid-closed loop insulin pump, and progress will continue as technology gets closer to making "artificial pancreas" pumps available to patients. There are also blunted responses of the counter-regulatory hormones meant to protect against hypoglycemia in patients with T1DM. Low- to moderate-intensity exercise generally results in hypoglycemia during exercise, while high-intensity exercises like sprinting, resistance training, or intense sports can lead to hyperglycemia during exercise. The hyperglycemia can be moderated by adjusting insulin dosing along with a light or moderate warm-up. It is important to note that the risk of hyperglycemia during intense exercise and/or with decreased insulin dosing to avoid hypoglycemia puts patients and athletes at an increased risk of ketosis with any activity. The risk of hypoglycemia may last up to 24 hours following a bout of exercise, putting a priority on monitoring and avoidance of nocturnal hypoglycemia, which can be severe and even fatal.

TABLE 9-3

SUGGESTED EXERCISE TRAINING PROTOCOL FOR PEOPLE WITH TYPE I DIABETES MELLITUS

VARIABLE	SUGGESTION
Program duration (months)	≥ 2
Frequency (days/week)	≥ 3
Type of training	Strength + HIIT
Session duration (minutes)	60 (35 of strength + 25 of HIIT)
Intensity	Vigorous (8 repetitions maximum* in strength and ~90% HR_{max} in HIIT)
Rest between high-intensity stimulus and strength exercises (minutes)	1
Total weekly duration (minutes)	≥ 180
Time between glucose measurements (minutes)	≤ 20

HIIT: high-intensity interval training; HR_{max}: maximum heart rate

*Maximum weight that participants could move 8 times with good technique: chest press, leg press, lateral pull down, leg extension, shoulder press, leg curl, and abdominal crunch

Glycemic goals for T1DM before exercise have been recommended to safely proceed with a lower risk of hypoglycemia in addition to avoiding hyperglycemia with slight variations between consensus statements (see Table 9-1).[24,29] The ADA suggests a fairly wide range of 90 to 250 mg/dL (5 to 13.9 mmol/L) while an international consensus considers a tighter goal range of 126 to 180 mg/dL (7 to 10 mmol/L), but both have similar and variable caveats for different individuals as noted in Figure 9-2. It is recommended to consume, or have available, additional carbs to maintain **euglycemia** during and after activity along with possible reductions in insulin dosing (Table 9-3).

Reducing basal insulin doses or basal insulin rates temporarily may be necessary to lessen the potential for delayed and/or nocturnal hypoglycemia along with healthy bedtime snacks. Due to the hyperglycemic effects of intense exercise, it has been suggested to supplement moderate exercise with sprints or resistance training to protect from hypoglycemic events. Some have advised making high-intensity anaerobic exercise primary modality in general for patients with T1DM to lower the risk of hypoglycemia.[29] Frequent blood glucose checks are also required to aid in insulin dosing and/or carb supplementation. CGM is very helpful and will continue to become a more commonly utilized tool, though there are limitations, especially for some intense and/or contact sports.

Athletes With Type I Diabetes Mellitus

There are not great data to suggest optimal goals for athletic performance, but one field study in adolescents suggested a clinically reasonable goal of about 108 to 144 mg/dL (6 to 8 mmol/L).[30]

For a patient or athlete in the field of practice or play, significant hyperglycemia, blood ketones, or recent episode of severe ("clinically significant") hypoglycemia (blood glucose < 54 mg/dL or 3 mmol/L) would be contraindication to initiating exercise or sport.[25,29]

Urgent Attention for Hypoglycemia

If an athletic trainer has an athlete experience hypoglycemia (low blood glucose of clinical relevance), he or she should be prepared for interventions performed according to the ADA recommendations based on expert opinion.[25] Symptoms of hypoglycemia may include tremor (shaking); heart racing or irregularity sensation (palpitations); anxiety; sweating; behavior or mental changes; and potentially seizure, coma, and/or death. Athletic trainers and exercise professionals should also be aware of signs exhibited by patients/clients with hypoglycemia including excessive sweating, which seems inappropriate, pallor (turning pale), and behavioral or cognitive changes as noted previously.

Pure glucose (15 to 20 gm, usually 3 to 5 glucose or dextrose tablets) is the preferred treatment for the conscious individuals with hypoglycemia (≤ 70 mg/dL [3.9 mmol/L]), although any form of carb that contains glucose may be used. Similar amounts of carbs are available in 4 oz of fruit juice, 5 oz of regular soda, 7 to 8 gummies or similar hard candy, or 1 tbsp of table sugar. High glycemic index sports drinks/gels may be a desirable option for athletes and should be on hand. Fifteen minutes after treatment, if SMBG +/- CGM shows continued hypoglycemia, the treatment should be repeated. Once blood glucose returns to normal, the individual should consume a meal or snack to prevent recurrence of hypoglycemia.

Glucagon should be administered if the patient is unable to consume carbs by mouth. Athletic trainers should be instructed on the use of glucagon kits, which are used to administer 1 mg either subcutaneously, intramuscularly, or intravenously once, depending on specific state guidelines concerning ability of athletic trainers to perform invasive procedures. This may be repeated every 15 to 20 minutes pending glycemic response.

Situations warranting emergency personnel include hypoglycemia associated with change in consciousness, seizure, and/or the need for use of glucagon

Conclusion

Physical activity and exercise prescriptions are a cornerstone in the comprehensive treatment plans for all individuals with DM. These interventions improve glycemic control and overall health. Personalized guidance and monitoring should vary by the type of diabetes, age of the patient/client, activity done or preferred, and presence of diabetes-related complications.

It remains a challenge for patients/athletes with T1DM to manage their disease optimally in order to garner the health benefits and/or optimize their participation in sporting events. It is critical for those patients/athletes and athletic trainers or exercise professionals to hone their skills in this regard to minimize the potential for the perilous complications of hypo- and hyperglycemia. It is important to have a basic understanding of the underling endocrinopathies involved with DM along with the nutritional needs, glycemic goals/monitoring, and insulin dosing strategies. It is also critical to be prepared for assisting with or managing those complications. A primary goal should be to personalize treatment and risk mitigation plans for all patients/athletes in collaboration with their health care team.

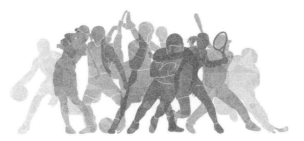

DEFINITIONS

Immunoglobulin: Any of a class of proteins present in the serum and cells of the immune system that function as antibodies

Secretagogues: A substance that promotes secretion

Endocrinopathies: A disease of an endocrine gland; a common medical term for a hormone problem

Euglycemia: Normal concentration of glucose in the blood; also called *normoglycemia*

REFERENCES

1. Ownby D. Exposure to dogs and cats in the first year of life and risk of allergic sensitization at 6 to 7 years of age. *J Am Med Assoc.* 2002;288(8):963.
2. Genuneit J. Exposure to farming environments in childhood and asthma and wheeze in rural populations: a systematic review with meta-analysis. *Pediatr Allergy Immunol.* 2012;23(6):509-518.
3. Waser M, Michels K, Bieli C, et al. Inverse association of farm milk consumption with asthma and allergy in rural and suburban populations across Europe. *Clin Exp Allergy.* 2007;37(5):661-670.
4. Penders J, Kummeling I, Thijs C. Infant antibiotic use and wheeze and asthma risk: a systematic review and meta-analysis. *Eur Respir J.* 2011;38(2):295-302.
5. Bager P, Melbye M, Rostgaard K, Stabell Benn C, Westergaard T. Mode of delivery and risk of allergic rhinitis and asthma. *J Allergy Clin Immunol.* 2003;111(1):51-56.
6. Silvers K, Frampton C, Wickens K, et al. Breastfeeding protects against current asthma up to 6 years of age. *J Pediatr.* 2012;160(6):991-996.e1.
7. Kresser C. Got allergies? Your microbes could be responsible. *Chriskesser.com.* https://chriskresser.com/got-allergies-your-microbes-could-be-responsible/. Published April 28, 2016. Accessed March 23, 2018.
8. Venter C, Laitinen K, Vlieg-Boerstra B. Nutritional aspects in diagnosis and management of food hypersensitivity-the dietitians role. *J Allergy (Cairo).* 2012;2012:269376.
9. Young E, Stoneham MD, Petruckevitch A, Barton J, Rona R. A population study of food intolerance. *Lancet.* 1994;343(8906):1127-1130.
10. Rona RJ, Keil T, Summers C, et al. The prevalence of food allergy: a meta-analysis. *J Allergy Clin Immunol.* 2007;120(3):638-646.
11. Pascual CY, Crespo JF, Perez PG, Esteban MM. Food allergy and intolerance in children and adolescents, an update. *Eur J Clin Nutr.* 2000;54 Suppl 1:S75-S78.

12. Jansen JJ, Kardinaal AF, Huijbers G, Vlieg-Boerstra BJ, Martens BP, Ockhuizen T. Prevalence of food allergy and intolerance in the adult Dutch population. *J Allergy Clin Immunol.* 1994;93(2):446-456.

13. Zuberbier T, Edenharter G, Worm M, et al. Prevalence of adverse reactions to food in Germany–a population study. *Allergy.* 2004;59(3):338-345.

14. Eggesbo M. The prevalence of CMA/CMPI in young children. *Allergy.* 2001;56:393-402.

15. Vlieg-Boerstra BJ, Bijleveld MA, van der Heide S, et al. Development and validation of challenge materials for double-blind, placebo-controlled food challenges in children. *J Allergy Clin Immunol.* 2004;113:341-346.

16. Osterballe M, Hansen TK, Mortz CG, Host A, Bindslev-Jensen C. The prevalence of food hypersensitivity in an unselected population of children and adults. *Pediatr Allergy Immunol.* 2005;16:567-573.

17. Roehr CC, Edenharter G, Reimann S, et al. Food allergy and non-allergic food hypersensitivity in children and adolescents. *Clin Exp Allergy.* 2004;34:1534-1541.

18. Petruláková M, Valík L. Food allergy and intolerance. *Acta Chimica Slovaca.* 2015;8(1):44-51.

19. Skyler JS, Bakris GL, Bonifacio E, et al. Differentiation of diabetes by pathophysiology, natural history, and prognosis. *Diabetes.* 2017;66(2):241-255.

20. Schwartz SS, Epstein S, Corkey BE, Grant SF, Gavin JR 3rd, Aguilar RB. The time is right for a new classification system for diabetes: rationale and implications of the B-cell-centric classification schema. *Diabetes Care.* 2016;39(2):179-186.

21. American Diabetes Association. Classification and diagnosis of diabetes. *Diabetes Care.* 2017;40(Suppl 1):S11-S24.

22. American Diabetes Association. Lifestyle management. *Diabetes Care.* 2017;40(Suppl 1):S33-S43.

23. Handelsman Y, Bloomgarden ZT, Grunberger G, et al. American Association of Clinical Endocrinologists and American College of Endocrinology Clinical Practice Guidelines for Developing a Diabetes Mellitus Comprehensive Care Plan—2015 Executive Summary. *Endocr Pract.* 2015;21(4):413-437.

24. Colberg SR, Sigal RJ, Yardley JE, et al. Physical activity/exercise and diabetes: a position statement of the American diabetes association. *Diabetes Care.* 2016;39(11):2065-2079.

25. American Diabetes Association. Glycemic targets. *Diabetes Care.* 2017;40(Suppl 1):S48-S56.

26. American Diabetes Association. Obesity management for the treatment of type 2 diabetes. *Diabetes Care.* 2017;40(Suppl 1):S57-S63.

27. American Diabetes Association. Pharmacologic approaches to glycemic treatment. *Diabetes Care.* 2017;40(Suppl. 1):S64-S74.

28. Garvey WT, Mechanick JI, Brett EM, et al. American Association of Clinical Endocrinologists and American College of Endocrinology Comprehensive Clinical Practice Guidelines for Medical Care of Patients with Obesity. *Endocr Pract.* 2016;22(Suppl 3):1-203.

29. Riddell MC, Gallen IW, Smart CE, et al. Exercise management in type 1 diabetes: a consensus statement. *Lancet Diabetes Endocrinol.* 2017;5(5):377-390.

30. Kelly D, Hamilton JK, Riddell MC. Blood glucose levels and performance in a sports camp for adolescents with type 1 diabetes mellitus: a field study. *Int J Pediatr.* 2010;2010:216167.

Conclusion

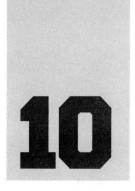

As we have seen several times in this text, nutrition research can be controversial, unclear, contradicting, manipulative, biased, and expensive. It is precisely those reasons that require a very calculated eye when deciphering what is truth, what is potential truth, and what is snake oil. What counts more than any other aspect of coaching athletes with regard to eating habits is consistency with a practitioners' recommendations. Attempting to source the next fad diet from the internet will only serve to obscure facts, conflate arguments toward validity, and confuse our athletes.

Practitioners would do well to take specific steps toward understanding future research or claims because good information will come out; the problem is it will be surrounded by a cloud of misinformation. First, practitioners should be able to identify the argument being made and what its specific claim is, as well as classifying what information, behavior, or results you would need to see in order to change your belief system based on this specific claim. From there, practitioners should be able to analyze the argument for or against a claim. Many aspects should be taken into account, such as quality of the research being done. Is it observational? Randomized? Large enough sample size? As we saw in the chapter on myths, it is fairly easy to manipulate data to seem compelling when really the results show nothing more than a very small change that is not statistically significant. The results may also be nothing more than correlation. In Figure 10-1, you can see that any data can be manipulated to show a positive correlation.

Clearly, US spending on science, space, and technology has no legitimate causation for increases in suicides by hanging, strangulation, and suffocation, but this chart can be manipulated with results to make it seem like they are connected. Obviously, this is an egregious example, but it goes to show what some researchers who may be desperate for continued funding may be willing to do in order to publish their work.

Amato D. *An Athletic Trainer's Guide
to Sports Nutrition (pp 159-160).*
© 2019 SLACK Incorporated.

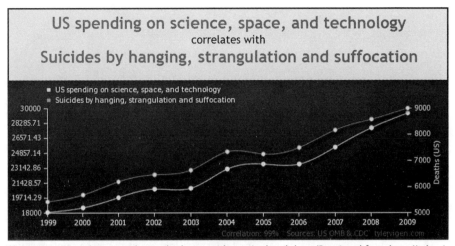

Figure 10-1. Correlation can be easily shown with manipulated data. (Reprinted from http://tylervigen.com/view_correlation?id=1597 via Creative Commons.)

Once you have gotten past the surface of a nutrition or health claim, it is time to really assess the validity. Is the claim supported by the evidence? Is that evidence realistic and presented logically? Furthermore, does the evidence of the claim go beyond the scope of what is presented? These are all pertinent questions to be asked when assessing anything new or different. Once you have exhausted your own research, you must remain skeptical. Continue to be skeptical of any new claim, especially ones that claim to be breakthroughs or magic fixes. There are so many new claims, research, fad diets, quick fixes, and promises made on a regular basis that it can be very difficult to discern what are good data and what are not. It is the responsibility of the practitioner to always be on top of the most recent research in order to best advise an athlete. Hopefully, this text will provide a broad-based explanation of pertinent mechanisms and important information for practitioners to extrapolate into real world situations. Individual situations require individual attention, something that all practitioners should recognize.

Financial
Disclosures

Mr. Damon Amato has no financial or proprietary interest in the materials presented herein.

Dr. Jennifer L. Gaudiani has no financial or proprietary interest in the materials presented herein.

Mr. John Kiefer has no financial or proprietary interest in the materials presented herein.

Dr. Karl Nadolsky has no financial or proprietary interest in the materials presented herein.

Dr. Stacy Sims has no financial or proprietary interest in the materials presented herein.

Index